"I could have shaved years off my suffering if this book had been available when my disease was active. If you're fighting addiction now, this book will enlighten you and make you realize you're not alone."

Paul,
Addict in recovery

"As a physician working with the problems of addiction, I strongly recommend this book. Prescription drug abuse has not received the attention it deserves. This book sheds light on an important and compelling issue."

David Smith, MD
President
American Society of Addiction Medicine

"An absolutely wonderful book for friends or family of anyone who's addicted to pills. After you read this, you'll no longer feel confused about prescription drug abuse and addiction. As a former addict, I also believe the book is must reading for addicts — if they're ready and willing to read it."

Terry,
Addict in recovery

"This book is a unique and valuable resource. *Prescription Drug Abuse: The Hidden Epidemic* is concise and easy to read, yet it's comprehensive, thoroughly researched and contains outstanding authoritative references."

Alan S. Hollister, MD, PhD
Associate Professor of Medicine
and Pharmacology,
University of Colorado

"This book fills a long-standing void — that of the need for education about the rampant abuse of prescription medication."

Jean Sheffield, Pharmacist
Texas Pharmacy Association

PRESCRIPTION DRUG ABUSE

The Hidden Epidemic

A Guide for Coping and Understanding

Rod Colvin

Addicus Books, Inc.
Omaha, Nebraska

An Addicus Nonfiction Book

10 9 8 7 6 5 4 3 2
ISBN # 1-886039-22-4

This book is not intended to serve as a substitute for a physician, nor does the author intend to give medical advice contrary to that of an attending physician.

Library of Congress Cataloging-in-Publication Data
Colvin, Rod.
   Prescription drug abuse : the hidden epidemic : a guide to coping and understanding / Rod Colvin.
      p. cm.
   "An Addicus nonfiction book."
   Includes bibliographic references (p.) and index.
   ISBN 1-886039-22-4 (pbk. : alk. paper)
      1. Medication abuse. 2. Medication abuse—United States.
I. Title.
RM146.5.C651995
362.29'9—dc20   95-10446
                                                                    CIP

Printed in United States of America.

*To the memory of those
we've lost to the hidden epidemic*

Table of Contents

Acknowledgments

I'd like to express my appreciation to the many people who gave interviews or provided other information which helped make this book possible.

First, a special thank you to the following people who generously lent time and expertise: Bonnie Wilford, Director, Pharmaceutical Policy Research Center, George Washington University; Phillip H. Cogan, Argus Health Systems, Inc.; Jeff Baldwin, PharmD, Associate Professor, University of Nebraska College of Pharmacy; Gary Holt, PhD, Professor Pharmacy, Northeast Louisiana University; Bill Ford, PhD.

The many others I wish to thank include: David Smith, MD, President, American Society Addiction Medicine; Robert L. DuPont, MD, former Director National Institute on Drug Abuse; Russell K. Portenoy, MD, Director, Analgesic Studies, Pain Service, Neurology Dept., Memorial Sloan-Kettering Cancer Center, New York; Alan Hollister, MD, University of Colorado Medical School; Brian Goldman, MD, University of Toronto, Toronto, Canada; David Joranson, Associate Director for Policy Studies, Pain Research Group, University of Wisconsin.

Sandra Bauer, Chairperson, California Controlled Substances Prescription Advisory Council; Deborah Hogan; Rick Seymour; Jody Gingery, Co-Chairperson Colorado Prescription Drug Abuse Task Force; John Duncan, Chief Agent, Oklahoma Bureau of Narcotics and Dangerous Drugs Control; Bill Couch, Drug Enforcement Administration; Linda McKaig and Janet Greenblatt, Substance Abuse & Mental Health Services Administration.

Audry Clayton and Leslie G. Aronovitz, General Accounting Office; John Eadie, Director, Division of Public Health Protection, New York Department of Health; James Egnot, MDM, MPH, New York Department of Health; Billy S. Allsbrook, Virginia State Police, Sgt. Ritch Wagner, Nebraska State Patrol; Bill Marcus, Assistant Attorney General, California; Sherry Green, Executive Director, National Alliance for Model State Drug Laws; Ronald Gershman, MD.

Patrick Dalton, Program Director, Addiction Institute; Betty Ferrell, RN, PhD, Associate Research Scientist Pain Management, City of Hope National Medical Center; Ed Polich, Director External Affairs, Whitby Pharmaceuticals, Inc./UCB Pharma; Margaret Crossen, McGrath Crossen & Associates; Steffie Woolhandler, MD, Harvard University Medical School; Thomas D. Wyatt, Executive Director National Association of State Controlled Substances Authorities; Carmon Catizone, Executive Director National Association of Boards of Pharmacy; Sidney H. Schnoll, MD, Chairman, Division of Substance Abuse, Medical College of Virginia.

Caroline Kearney Hershfeld, Co-Founder Benzodiazepines Anonymous; Terence Gorski, Relapse Prevention Specialist; Scott Nelson, Manager Public Affairs, DuPont-Merck Pharmaceuticals; Dixon Arnett, Executive Director, Medical Board of California; Len Yesh, Tennessee Alcohol and Drug Association; David Mee-Lee, MD, Castle Medical Center, Honolulu; Le Clair Bissel, MD; Shiela Blume, MD, South Oaks Hospital, Amityville, New York; David Gastfriend, MD, Massachusetts General Hospital, Boston; Chris Kasser, MD; Paul Somsky, MD; Joanne Schuler, Special Agent, Tennessee Bureau of Investigation; Jeff Trewitt, Vice President for Communications, Pharmaceutical Research and Manufacturers of America. Bob Lutz, Director of Business Planning and Development, Knoll Pharmaceuticals; Jeff Newton, Director Media Relations, Eli Lilly & Co.; Susan Obrebski, Librarian, National Association of Chain Drug Stores; Mitch Rothholtz, American Pharmaceutical Association; William P. Egherman, MD, Craig Alan Sinkinson, MD, Greg Wokersien, CME-TV, Inc., Michael Moy, Chief,

Drug Operations Sections, Drug Enforcement Administration
(DEA), Washington, D.C.

National Council on Patient Education and Information;
Alcoholics Anonymous; Narcotics Anonymous.

I would especially like to thank those who shared their
personal stories of recovery. They are identified by first
names only: Michelle Z., Margaret P., Justin L., Barbara B.,
Don A., Nancy N., Terry S. and Jeff S.

Finally a word of warm thanks to my friends — Tom
McFarland, Susan Adams, Rosalea Maher, Harry Thiele, Betty
Wright, David Zaloudek, Harriett Knake, Gregg Olsen, Jeff
Hutton and Shelton Hendricks — whose help and encourage-
ment made this book possible.

Introduction

The purpose for this book is twofold: to help individuals and families battling prescription drug abuse or addiction and to inform others about this serious national problem.

My interest in prescription drug abuse results from the loss of my brother, Randy. His sudden death in 1988, at age 35, was, in large part, due to his years of dependency on prescription drugs — tranquilizers and sedatives. Now, having recovered from the loss, I've had more time to clearly reflect on my family's experience with his dependency.

Randy became dependent on tranquilizers in his early 20s, when a psychiatrist first prescribed them for anxiety. His drug abuse escalated over the years. Our family struggled to both help him and cope with what was clearly addiction. Although at the time, we didn't see it as addiction — after all, the drugs were prescriptions.

I remember my stunned disbelief at seeing his drugs of choice coming from prescriptions — written by physicians, filled at local pharmacies. He could get virtually any drug he wanted, any time he wanted it. The medical establishment, with every good intention of helping, was being manipulated again and again. Although I considered my brother responsible for his behavior, I was also disturbed by the vulnerability of the medical community. Still, we coped and hoped things would get better. Unfortunately, the situation did not improve.

Ironically, the end came on October 19, my brother's birthday. He had also just finished his college degree in business, and had been drug free for nearly a year. The two of us had planned to make his birthday dinner a celebration. However, the celebration never came to pass.

Around mid-afternoon, I received a call from a local hospital, saying my brother had been brought in by rescue squad and that he was in critical condition. My heart pounding, I raced to the hospital, but it was too late. He'd been pronounced dead on arrival, the nurses told me.

Later, as I pieced together the last hours of my brother's life, I learned that he had relapsed. Although he had not overdosed, he apparently had taken tranquilizers along with alcohol. His physician told me that he likely suffered vertricular tachycardia, a fatal arrythmia, during which the heart flutters, then fails.

In spite of all the years of trying to help Randy, trying to save him, the worst had still happened. He died. His battle, my family's battle with prescription drug abuse was over. We had lost.

Now, other families fight the same battles. And they, like my family, are embarrassed by addiction and guard the "family secret." They suffer alone in silence and in shame. As public awareness stays locked on the war against illegal drugs, prescription drug abuse, misuse and addiction go misunderstood and under-reported.

This hidden epidemic demands attention. Solutions exist. However, there are no quick fixes, no easy answers; it is a multifaceted problem. And, one of the most serious dangers is imposing any restrictions which would impede the prescribing of narcotics to those who are seriously ill or suffering legitimate pain.

Still, until curbing prescription drug diversion is a priority, abuse will continue. The economic toll, but more importantly, the toll on human life, will be staggering.

PART ONE

The Hidden Epidemic

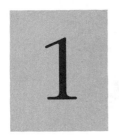

1 Prescription Drug Abuse, Addiction, Misuse

S omewhere at this very moment, a mother agonizes as her
adult son, intoxicated on tranquilizers, destroys yet another family gathering.

Elsewhere, a young man is writing out his own sedative
prescription on a pad he's stolen from a doctor's office. And
somewhere within the walls of a respected hospital, a nurse
is shooting Demerol into her own veins, while her patient
unknowingly gets an injection of saline solution. The case
scenarios go on and on. Legions of Americans are abusing
prescription drugs.

In fact, chances are you know someone who is abusing
pharmaceuticals. Maybe it's your spouse, a relative, a friend
or a casual acquaintance. Maybe it's you. It's possible that you
don't even realize the use has shifted from therapeutic to
abusive.

Prescription drug abuse is often difficult to recognize. The
abuse is usually an intensely private affair between the abuser
and a bottle of pills. And, the pill-taker is not subject to the
social stigma associated with the shadowy world of street-
drug dealing.

Abuse, when it becomes addiction, can be especially confusing for friends and family of the one who's dependent.

You assume that a medical need for the medication exists or the drugs would not have been prescribed. These are legal medications — not alcohol, not a substance to be smoked or snorted. Yet you know the user is escalating doses and using the medication inappropriately. What will you do? What can you do? Do you call the prescribing doctor and report the medication abuse? Do you confront the abuser? You may already know you can't reason with a person when he or she is chemically affected. Maybe you're hoping the problem will get better. Perhaps everything will work out in the end.

And you may be correct. The prescription drug abuser you know might decide to "pull up the boot straps" and get straight. Many people are able to do that, whether it be alcohol or pills they're using. But, what about the other possibility...that of the abuser spiraling downward, deeper into abuse and addiction. Then what?

These are just some of the stubborn questions facing families as this epidemic of prescription drug abuse continues. If your family is fortunate, the abuser will change. If not, realize that the abuser's behavior is taking an emotional toll on the entire family. No one escapes it.

You might be well served by first educating yourself about the dynamics of addiction and how it affects users and their families. Education — rather than guess work — can be your first line of defense.

On a broader scale, public education is key to curbing this serious national problem. How serious is it? This question calls for data, but citing statistics on the numbers of Americans abusing or diverting pharmaceuticals is difficult, at best. No reliable statistics exist on the extent of diversion from legitimate prescribers. And, opinions among experts vary, with some quantifying the problem as "minimal," while others describe it as "widespread," insisting that the numbers that do appear in scientific studies are far too low.

Nonetheless, according to the National Household Survey on Drug Abuse in 1993, eight million Americans, reported having used prescription drugs — stimulants, sedatives, tran-

Table 1. Most Frequently Abused Substances in the United States in 1993, by numbers of persons.

(People aged 12 and over reporting use of a substance within the last year)

Drug Class	Number of Persons Abusing
Illicit Drug Abuse	**24,400,000**
Marijuana and Hashish	18,600,000
Cocaine	4,500,000
Crack	996,000
Inhalants	2,100,000
LSD, Hallucinogens	2,400,000
Heroin	245,000
Prescription Drug Abuse	**7,900,000**
Stimulants	2,400,000
Analgesics	4,600,000
Tranquilizers	2,500,000
Sedatives	1,600,000
Alcohol (Heavy Drinking)	**138,000,000**
Cigarettes	**61,000,000**
Smokeless Tobacco	8,200,000
Anabolic Steroids	134,000

Numbers may not total the sum at the top of categories since individuals may have reported the use of more than one substance.

Source: From "Preliminary Estimates from the 1993 National Household Survey on Drug Abuse" Substance Abuse & Mental Health Services Administration (SAMHSA), 1993. U.S. Department of Health and Human Services, Report 7, p. 48.

quilizers or analgesics — for nonmedical purposes (See Table 1).

In addition, data from the Substance Abuse and Mental Health Services Administration show that 30% to 50% of those drugs listed by patients treated for misuse or overdose in hospital emergency rooms were prescription drugs. In fact, prescription drug overdoses outnumbered heroin overdoses by a ratio of 6:1. It's important to note, however, that the emergency room data likely inflate abuse statistics since suicide attempts are included.

Yet another measure of the problem is reflected by a 1991 national survey of drug treatment facilities. The survey, conducted for the National Institute on Drug Abuse, found that the drug of choice among 9.4% of the patients was a "prescription drug."

The Drug Enforcement Administration (DEA) reports that 12 of the top 20 abused controlled substances in the United States are prescription drugs (See Table 2). Further, the agency estimates that as many as tens of millions of drug doses may be diverted annually for the purpose of abuse. Acquisition of the drugs can occur anywhere between the point of manufacture and the retail or hospital level.

Prescription drug abuse can be classified into several, general categories: 1) abuse, 2) addiction or dependency, and 3) misuse. Keep in mind that boundaries between these categories can blur, with people shifting from one group into another.

Another serious element of prescription drug diversion, black market or street sales, is covered in Chapter Eight.

Prescription Drug Abuse

In *The Pharmacological Basis of Therapeutics*, Jerome Jaffe defines drug abuse as "the use, usually by self-administration, of any drug in a manner that deviates from the approved medical use or social patterns within a given culture. The term conveys the notion of social disapproval, and it is not necessarily descriptive of any particular pattern of drug use or its potential adverse consequences."

Table 2. Top 20 Most Abused Controlled Substances

1. Cocaine
2. Heroin
3. Marijuana
4. Alprazolam (*Xanax*)
5. Diazepam (*Valium*)
6. Lorazepam (*Ativan*)
7. Clonazepam (*Klonopin*)
8. Methamphetamine
9. Codeine combinations
10. Unspecified benzodiazepines
11. D-Propoxyphene (*Darvon, Darvocet*)
12. PCP & PCP combinations
13. Hydrocodone (*Vicodin, Lorcet, Lortab*)
14. Amphetamine
15. Hashish
16. Temazepam (*Restoril*)
17. Oxycodone (*Percodan, Percocet, Tylox, Roxicodone*)
18. LSD
19. Chlordiazepoxide (*Librium, Libritabs*)
20. Methadone

Source: From "Drug Abuse Warning Network Emergency Room Data" Drug Enforcement Administration, Office of Diversion Control, 1993, p. 2-7.

Abused substances may be obtained from any number of sources — by prescriptions, from a friend, over-the-counter, or through the illicit market. It's a common misconception that the use must occur daily to indicate abuse — the pattern of use may be occasional or habitual.

Commonly Abused Opioids, Stimulants and Sedatives

Opioids and narcotic analgesics are typically prescribed to relieve acute or chronic pain such as that from cancer or surgery. For acute pain, opioids are normally used only for short periods — less than 30 days. Opioids may be taken orally or by injection. Common **opioids** include:

Darvocet	Darvon
Demerol	Dilaudid
Drugs with Codeine	Methadone
Morphine	Percocet
Percodan	Roxicet
Roxiprin	Tussionex
Vicodin	

Stimulants are central nervous system stimulants which increase mental alertness, decrease fatigue and produce a sense of well-being. These drugs are often prescribed for attention deficit disorder (hyperactivity) and narcolepsy:

Ritalin

Dexedrine

Cyclert

Ritalin, although a stimulant, has a calming effect on children diagnosed with hyperactivity by stimulating nerves which slow down other overactive nerves. Other stiumlants often used to suppress appetite include: Fastin, Dexedrine, Didrex, Preludin, Plegine and Tenuate.

Sedatives and hypnotics such as barbiturates and benzodiazepines depress the central nervous system and are frequently used to treat anxiety, panic disorder or insomnia.

Sedatives (benzodiazepines) often prescribed for daytime use:

Ativan	Klonopin
Librium	Serax
Tranxene	Valium
Xanax	

Benzodiazepines frequently used for nighttime insomnia:

Dalmane	Doral and Prosom
Halcion	Restoril

According to the Drug Abuse Warning Network, analysis of 1993 hospital emergency room data showed that 69% of the licit drugs misused by patients were benzodiazepines; these drugs were often used in combination with alcohol. Most deaths from benzodiazepines are caused by combined use with alcohol.

Debate continues in the medical community over the safe, long-term use of benzodiazepines, since build up of tolerance is often rapid and severe withdrawal can occur if these drugs are stopped abruptly. The debate prompted the American Psychiatric Association to issue a statement claiming, "Physiological dependence on benzodiazepines...can develop with therapeutic doses. Duration of treatment determines the onset of dependence...clinically significant dependence usually does not appear before four months of such daily dosing. Dependence may develop sooner when higher antipanic doses are taken daily."

Anyone who has used benzodiazepines over an extended period of time, should never stop taking the drug on his or her own. These individuals should be medically supervised so that withdrawal can be managed as the patient is tapered off the drug. Medically unsupervised withdrawal can be severe, leading to delirium, fever, seizures, coma and even death.

Another symptom of withdrawal is "symptom rebound" — an intensified return of the original symptoms, such as insomnia or anxiety, for which the drug was first prescribed. This rebound is often misinterpreted by patients as a recurrence of anxiety.

Some of the controversy surrounding the use of benzodiazepines has resulted from the drug's misuse by chemically dependent patients. "Patients who have a current or past history of chemical dependence, including heavy alcohol and the current or past use abuse of drugs and/or alcohol, are poor candidates for use of benzodiazepines in the treatment of anxiety," states Robert L. DuPont, MD, former Director of the National Institute on Drug Abuse. "Anyone who has used illicit drugs repeatedly over a period of months or years, and anyone who drinks more than a few drinks of alcohol a week, should use benzodiazepines with extreme caution, if at all" (See Table 3).

Drug Addiction

Addiction may be defined as a pattern of compulsive drug use characterized by a continued craving for drugs and the need to use these drugs for psychological effects or mood alterations. Many abusers find that they need to use drugs to feel "normal." The user exhibits drug-seeking behavior and is often preoccupied with using and obtaining the drugs of choice. These substances may be obtained through legal or illegal channels (See Table 4).

The American Society of Addiction Medicine considers addiction "a disease process characterized by the continued use of a specific psychoactive substance despite physical, psychological or social harm."

Studies show that between 10% and 16% of the American population is identified as being chemically dependent at some point during their lifetimes. Seven million Americans are in recovery from addictive diseases.

Distinguishing Physiological Dependence from Addiction

Often confused with addiction is "physiological dependence," which is a result of the body's adaptation to a drug used over a period of time to treat a medical disorder. For example, a patient taking pain medication for several weeks would likely develop some degree of tolerance to the drug, and would have withdrawal symptoms if the drug was stopped abruptly. Abstinence symptoms could include anxiety, irritability, chills alternating with hot flashes, salivation, nausea, or abdominal cramps. This syndrome, however, is not addiction.

With physiological dependence, the patient can quit the drug, usually gradually, with medical supervision and without admission into a drug treatment program. (See Table 5).

"A decade ago, it was widely believed that virtually anyone who took psychoactive drugs was a likely candidate for

---

Table 3. Benzodiazepine Checklist

Questions to consider for long-term benzodiazepine prescriptions:

1. **Diagnosis and response to treatment**
   Does the patient have a clear-cut diagnosis and does the patient respond favorably to the use of the benzodiazepines?

2. **Use of psychotropic substances**
   Is the patient's use of alcohol and other substances legal and sensible? Does the patient avoid all use of illegal drugs? Is the benzodiazepine dose reasonable? Is the use of other prescribed drugs medically reasonable?

3. **Toxic behavior**
   Is the patient free of slurred speech, accidents, or other problems that may be associated with excessive or inappropriate use of any prescribed or nonprescribed psychoactive substance?

4. **Family monitor**
   Does a family member confirm that the patient's use of the benzodiazepines is both sensible and helpful and that the patient does not abuse alcohol or use illegal substances?

A "no" answer to any of these questions suggests the need to discontinue benzodiazepines. A "yes" to all four questions supports continuation of benzodiazepine prescriptions if that is the shared conclusion of patient and physician. The standard to be met: Is this treatment clearly in the patient's best interest?

Source: From "Benzodiazepines, addiction and public policy" by Robert L. DuPont, MD, 1993, *New Jersey Medicine*, 90:824-826. Copyright 1993 by *New Jersey Medicine*. Reprinted by permission.

---

dependency. But that thinking has changed," said Bonnie Wilford, Director, Pharmaceutical Policy Research Center, George Washington University, which analyzes national drug use trends. "Our change of thought has come about as a result of our increased knowledge about addiction. Perhaps 7 out of 10 people could take tranquilizers, for example, for a

Table 4. Distinguishing Medical Substance Use from Nonmedical Substance Use

	Medical Use	Nonmedical Use
Intent	To treat diagnosed illness	To alter mood
Effect	Makes life of user better	Makes life of user worse
Pattern	Steady and sensible	Chaotic and high dose
Legality	Legal	Illegal (except alcohol or tobacco use by adults)
Control	Shared with physician	Self-controlled

Source: From "Benzodiazepines, addiction and public policy" by Robert L. DuPont, MD, 1993, *New Jersey Medicine*, 90:824-826. Copyright 1993 by *New Jersey Medicine*. Reprinted by permission.

very long time and not progress to addiction. But those who do become addicted likely have a pre-existing addictive disorder, such as alcoholism. The difficulty is a doctor doesn't always know which patients this will be." Those considered to be at increased risk of addiction have family histories of addiction or have such problems as depression, hyperactivity, chronic pain syndromes or obesity. Other groups at increased risk are medical professionals, drug abusers, former addicts, alcoholics and smokers. Additionally, extreme stress such as family tragedy, death or divorce may precipitate abusive drug use.

Prescription Drug Misuse

If you're taking a prescription drug now, chances are one in two that you're taking it incorrectly. According to the National Council on Patient Information and Education, 1.7 billion prescriptions are dispensed annually in the United States, and more than 50% of these prescriptions are used incorrectly. Drug misusers, those people unintentionally using drugs improperly with the intent of getting therapeutic benefit, make up the largest, yet most hidden group.

Misuse or noncompliance is a major health problem in the United States, resulting in 125,000 deaths annually and adding $20 billion to annual health care costs. Misuse includes many scenarios, ranging from the health professional who misprescribes to the patient who stops taking a medication or who may be exchanging drugs with family members or friends.

Table 5. The distinction between addiction and physiological dependence

Addiction

- Loss of control
- Continued use despite problems caused by use
- Denial
- Relapse
- A complex, biobehavioral, lifelong, malignant problem
- Limited to chemically dependent people
- Not a complication of medical treatment unless there is a prior history of chemical dependence
- Best treated by specific chemical dependence treatment

Physiological dependence

- A cellular adaptation to presence of a substance
- Withdrawal symptoms on abrupt discontinuation
- Not associated with relapse
- A benign, temporary problem
- Common to many substances used in medicine including steroids, anti-depressants, anti-epilepsy, and anti-hypertensive medicines
- Best treated by gradual dose reduction

Source: From "Benzodiazepines, addiction and public policy" by Robert L. DuPont, MD, 1993, *New Jersey Medicine*, 90:824-826. Copyright 1993 by *New Jersey Medicine*. Reprinted by permission.

The use of some prescription drugs in combination with alcohol can constitute misuse that can be serious and potentially lethal. Even though a drinker may have developed tolerance to the sedative effects of alcohol, he or she will not have developed a tolerance for the alcohol's depressing effects on the respiratory system. The combination of alcohol and tranquilizers or sedatives can create further cardio-respiratory depression and lead to death.

Factors contributing to misuse

- Poor patient/provider communication (Most office visits last 15 minutes or less)
- Use of multiple medicines with similar effects
- Use of multiple providers
- Inability to take the medication as prescribed
- Deliberate noncompliance
- Altered drug action and response due to advancing age or the effects of other drugs

Misuse of medications has serious consequences including:

- Addiction
- Prolonged illness
- Avoidable side effects
- Drug interactions
- Increased hospitalization
- Absences from work
- Over-utilization of health care services
- Death

How to Avoid the Misuse of Medications

Ask questions, make sure you understand how the medication works.

Tell your physician and pharmacist:

- The names of all medicine you are taking, including all nonprescription medications you are or might consider taking

- Problems you are having or have had with any medications
- Any allergies you have, including allergy to any medicines
- If you are or think you are pregnant or if you are breast feeding

Overmedication and undermedication are also considered forms of misuse. Overmedication is defined as the inappropriate use of a drug at dosages higher than those needed to treat an illness. Undermedication occurs when a patient takes less than the prescribed dose or takes it infrequently.

Schedule of Controlled Substances

Why does the federal government rank controlled substances by schedule? Recognizing the abuse potential of many medications, the Congress enacted the Controlled Substances Act in 1970 to better regulate the manufacture, distribution and dispensing of controlled substances. The Act divides into five schedules those drugs known to have potential for physical or psychological harm, based on their potential for abuse, accepted medical use and accepted safety under medical supervision.

Schedule I drugs, such as heroin, have a high potential for abuse, no generally accepted medical use in the United States and are not available through legal means. Schedules II through V contain drugs with accepted medical uses but some abuse potential. Schedule II pharmaceuticals are the most likely to be abused, Schedule V the least.

The Drug Enforcement Administration monitors the registration, record-keeping and drug security of those handling and receiving controlled substances.

Examples from the five categories of controlled substances:

Schedule I

Heroin   Marijuana

LSD   Peyote

Mescaline

Phenclyclidine (PCP)

MDA

Psilocybin

Methaqualone
(formerly Quaalude)

MDMA ("Ecstasy")

Schedule II

High potential for abuse. Use may lead to severe physical or psychological dependence. Prescriptions must be written in ink, or typewritten and signed by the practitioner. Verbal prescriptions must be confirmed in writing within 72 hours, and may be given only in a genuine emergency. No refills are permitted.

Alfentanil (*Alfenta*)

Amphetamine (*Dexedrine*)

Cocaine

Hydromorphone
(*Dilaudid*)

Levorphanol
(*Levo-Dromoran*)

Methadone (*Dolophine*)

Meperidine (*Demerol*)

Morphine (*MS Contin,
Oramorph, Roxanol*, others)

Oxycodone (*Percodan,
Percocet, Tylox, Roxicodone*)

Pentobarbital (*Nembutal*)

Secobarbital (*Seconal*)

Amobarbital (*Amytal*)

Codeine

Fentanyl (*Sublimaze,
Duragesic*)
Glutethimide

Levomethadyl
(*ORLAAM*)

Marinol (*Dronabinol*)

Methamphetamine
(*Desoxyn*)

Methylphenidate
(*Ritalin*)

Opium (*Pantopon*)

Oxymorphone
(*Numorphan*)

Phenmetrazine (*Preludin*)

Sufentanil (*Sufenta*)

Schedule III

Some potential for abuse. May lead to low-to-moderate physical dependence or high psychological dependence. Prescriptions may be oral or written. Up to five renewals are permitted within six months.

Anabolic steroids (numerous products such as *Halotestin, Anadrol, Winstrol, Oxandrin, Durabolin*)

Benzphetamine (*Didrex*)

Butalbital (with aspirin and caffeine — *Fiorinal, Fiorgen, Isollyl*)

Butabarbital (*Butisol*)

Camphorated tincture of opium (*Paregoric*)

Codeine (low doses combined with non-narcotic medications such as *Tylenol, Phenaphen*, Aspirin, *Empirin, Soma* compound)

Hydrocodone (with acetaminophen — *Lorcet, Vicodin*; with Aspirin — *Lortab*; with chlorpheniramine — *Tussionex*)

Methyprylon (*Noludar*)

Nalorphine

Phendimetrazine (*Plegine*)

Testosterone

Schedule IV

Lower potential for abuse. Use may lead to limited physical or psychological dependence. Prescriptions may be oral or written. Up to five refills are permitted within six months.

Alprazolam (*Xanax*)	Chloral Hydrate (*Nortec*)
Chlordiazepoxide (*Librium, Libritabs*)	Clonazepam (*Klonopin*)
Clorazepate (*Tranxene*)	Diazepam (*Valium, Valrelease*)
Ethchlorvynol (*Placidyl*)	Flurazepam (*Dalmane*)

Lorazepam (*Ativan*)   Mephobarbital (*Mebaral*)

Meprobamate (*Equinil, Miltown*)   Midazolam (*Versed*)

Oxazepam (*Serax*)   Pemoline (*Cyclert*)

Pentazocine (*Talwin*)   Phenobarbital (*Luminal*)

Phentermine (*Fastin*)   Prazepam (*Centrax*)

Propoxyphene (*Darvon, Darvocet*)   Quazepam (*Doral*)

Temazepam (*Restoril*)   Triazolam (*Halcion*)

Schedule V

Subject to state and local regulation. Abuse potential is low; addictive medication is often combined with nonaddicting medicines to reduce abuse potential. A prescription may not be required.

Codeine   (in low doses combined with non-narcotic medications such as *Actifed, Novahistine DH, Terpin Hydrate, Ambenyl, Prometh, Tuss-Organidin, Phenergan, Dihistine DH, Dimetane-DC, Robitussin A-C, Cheracol*)

Buprenorphine (*Buprenex*)

Diphenoxylate (*Lomotil*)

2 The Elderly — at Risk for Misuse

I f you're a senior citizen or if you have parents or grandparents who are, take note. The nation's elderly are at high risk for drug misuse. Grandmothers and grandfathers are showing up in emergency rooms, overdosed on such pills as Valium, Xanax and other tranquilizers.

People 65 and older make up 13% of the US population, yet they take 30% of all prescription drugs sold in the United States. Millions of seniors take up to six medications daily. If care is not taken to see that drugs work safely together, the results can be harmful. Each year, such misuse among the elderly accounts for more than 9 million adverse drug reactions and 245,000 hospitalizations; 25% of nursing home admissions occur annually as a result of seniors' inability to use medicines safely.

In addition to inappropriate mixing of medications, seniors metabolize drugs differently than younger people. As normal changes in body makeup occur, the percent of water and lean tissue decreases as fat increases. Also, the kidneys and liver can begin to function less efficiently. Both these factors affect the time a drug stays in the body and the amount absorbed by body tissues.

Harvard Study on Harmful Medications for the Elderly

In the first national study of its kind, researchers at Harvard University reported in 1994 that 28% of the nation's senior citizens, nearly 7 million people, are taking prescribed drugs considered dangerous to their health. Experts say the study only scratches the surface, that one-half to two-thirds of senior citizens, living in communities, are being prescribed drugs that are doing unnecessary harm to them (See Table 6).

What is the biggest risk factor for the elderly in taking medications? "I think taking sedatives or sleeping pills is the most dangerous thing for elderly people," said Dr. Steffie Woolhandler, co-author of the study. "The drugs don't wear off by morning, leaving senior citizens sleepy and confused and prone to falling and hip fractures."

Woolhandler attributes part of the problem to physicians' misprescribing. "I'm a medical educator at Harvard, so speaking as an insider, I must say the education for young physicians about drug use is abysmal," she said. "We do not do a very good job teaching about drug therapy to medical students. I don't think I'm doctor bashing when I acknowledge that we medical educators need to do a better job of teaching physicians about medications."

Another facet of the problem — elderly patients may be seeing multiple physicians, getting different medications from each doctor and not reporting it. "That is very common in this age group," explains Bonnie Wilford, Director Pharmaceutical Policy Research, George Washington University. "The elderly are also very poor at reporting any alcohol use — they're ashamed of it."

A case in point…a 62-year-old California woman who had fallen and broken her hip. The hospital staff was unaware that the woman had been mixing Valium with wine and had become chemically dependent. The combination of chemicals caused her fall. "On the fourth day after her hip surgery, she started having very serious withdrawal and withdrawal delirium," reported Dr. David Smith of San Francisco, President of the American Society of Addiction Medicine. "It's a substantial

Table 6. Drugs to Avoid if You're Over 65

Tranquilizers, Sleeping Aids
Diazepam (*Valium*), tranquilizer. Addictive and too long-acting.

Chlordiazepoxide (*Librium, Librax*), tranquilizer. May cause falls.

Flurazepam (*Dalmane*), sleeping aid. May cause falls.

Meprobamate (*Miltown, Deprol, Equagesic, Equanil*), tranquilizer. May cause falls.

Pentobarbitol (*Nembutal*), sedative. Addictive.

Secobarbitol (*Seconal*), Addictive.

Anti-depressants
Amitriptyline (*Elavil, Endep, Etrafon, Limbitrol, Triavil*), often causes inability to urinate, dizziness and drowsiness.

Arthritis Drugs
Indomethacin (*Indocin*). Can cause confusion, headaches.

Phenylbutazone (*Butazolidin*). Risk of bone marrow toxicity.

Diabetes Drugs
Chlorpropramide (*Diabinese*). Can cause dangerous fluid retention.

Pain Relievers
Propoxyphene (*Darvon Compound, Darvocet, Wygesic*). Addictive and little more effective than asprin.

Pentazocine. (*Talwin*). Addictive.

Dementia Treatments
Cyclandelate. Not shown to be effective

Isoxsuprine. Not shown to be effective.

Blood Thinners
Dipyidamole, (*Persantine*). Except inpatients with artificial heart valves, not shown effective.

Muscle Relaxants, Spasm Relievers
Cyclobenzaprine (*Flexeril*). Can cause dizziness, drowsiness, fainting.

Orphenidrine (*Norflex, Norgesic*). Can cause dizziness, drowsiness, fainting.

Methocarbamol (*Robaxin*). May cause dizziness or drowsiness.

Carisoprodol (*Soma*). Potential for central nervous system toxicity.

Anti-Nausea, Anti-Vomiting Drugs
Trimethobenzamide (*Tigan*). May cause drowsiness, dizziness and other reactions.

Anti-Hypertensives
Propranolol (*Inderal*). Feeling slowed mentally and physically.

Methyldopa (*Aldoril, Aldomet*). Feeling slowed mentally and physically.

Reserpine (*Regroton, Hydropres*). Depression.

Source: From "Inappropriate Drug Prescribing for the Community-Dwelling Elderly," by Sharon M. Wilson, David U. Himmelstein and Steffie Woolhandler, 1994, *Journal of the American Medical Association*, 272: 292-296. (Agency for Health Care Policy and Research) Copyright 1994 by *Journal of the American Medical Association*. Reprinted by permission.

problem in the elderly. Fifty percent of delirium in the elderly in hospitals is related to the side effects of prescription drugs." Confusion, slurred speech and memory loss are also side effects.

Statistics from nursing homes are also disturbing; one study, conducted by W.A. Ray and published in 1987 by the *New England Journal of Medicine* showed that 14% of hip fractures are attributed to the adverse effects of psychotropic drugs. If you have a relative in a nursing home, once or twice a year, ask the staff for a medical review of all drugs being prescribed.

Brown Bag Days

What can you do to prevent dangerous drug misuse for an elderly person? Participate in a "brown bag day." At least once a year, dump all medications in a brown bag and take it to a doctor or pharmacist for evaluation. The process should be repeated whenever a new drug is added. It's recommended that senior citizens have all medications filled at one pharmacy.

Among the common problems discovered during medicine reviews: medications are duplicated, with serious potential for overdose; inappropriate drug interactions; patient confusion over drugs with similar names; over/under-utilization when the patient has not understood the instructions.

Examples of Questions Asked by Medicine Reviewers

1. Do you have any medicine allergies?
2. What medical problem are you treating with this medicine?
3. How long have you been taking this medicine?
4. How long has it been since you visited the physician who prescribed this medication?
5. Is the medicine in the original container?
6. What is the purpose of this medication?

7. How are you supposed to take this medication — how much, how often?

8. What is your daily routine for taking the medicine?

9. Do you have any side effects from this medication?

10. What non-prescription medicines do you take? Why? When?

By the year 2000, the US Department of Health and Human Services hopes to increase to 75% the proportion of health care providers who conduct medicine reviews with older patients.

For information on setting up community "Brown Bag Days," write:

The National Council on Patient Information
    and Education (NCPIE)
666 11th Street, Suite 810
Washington, DC 20001

3   *Pain Management*

Many experts agree that legitimate pain in the United States is undermedicated. Pain management has come under much scrutiny, and fortunately, strides have been made in bringing relief to those suffering serious pain. In discussing the abuse of controlled substances, it's critical that high dosages of narcotics, often needed in the treatment of legitimate pain, not be confused with drug abuse.

"In the past few years we've tried to focus on improving pain management because we know that for the past several decades pain has not been well controlled," according to Betty R. Ferrell, RN, PhD, associate research scientist on pain management, City of Hope National Medical Center, Duarte, California. "Federal guidelines estimate that as many as half of the 13 million people who have surgery receive inadequate pain management. It's also estimated that as many as 80% of cancer patients do not receive adequate medication for pain."

As a result of these statistics, research is ongoing and new federal guidelines for pain management have been issued by the US Department of Health and Human Services. One of the main barriers to effective pain management, according to the guidelines, is fear of addiction.

"Unfortunately, the 'Just say no to drugs' campaign has had a negative impact on pain management. For example, when we talk to cancer patients about pain control, they are afraid they'll become drug addicts," Ferrell explains. "Several published research studies tell us that less than 1% of hospitalized medical inpatients receiving medical care for legitimate, acute pain become addicted. Yet many of these patients will be afraid they'll become addicted. Many patients who had surgery yesterday and who are in pain, are afraid to take pain medication. (The statistics may be different for certain groups of patients with chronic, nonmalignant pain.)

"One of the public awareness problems occurs when we hear about a celebrity who's addicted to prescription drugs. We think we're all candidates for such addiction; however, these celebrities usually had a history of alcoholism or addiction. And it is those patients who do have a history of substance abuse who can become addicted to their medication.

"Even terminal cancer patients, who need serious pain management, are often afraid of becoming 'junkies.' We've had parents whose children are dying with cancer, and even then we've had parents say 'my son is not going to die a junkie so I'm not going to give him that pain medication.' Children have had to talk parents into giving them their medication. So we have to explain to the parents the difference between drug addiction and physiological dependence. In the latter case, if the patient should eventually come off the pain medication, it would be done gradually with medical supervision; otherwise, the patient would have withdrawal."

At the University of Wisconsin, David Joranson, Associate Director for Policy Studies with the Pain Research Group, reports that patients' and doctors' expectations for effective pain management is much higher than in years before. "It's essential that we evaluate the barriers to effective pain relief. It's important to understand the role of opioid analgesics — they are the mainstay in the treatment of acute pain. Consumers should talk to care givers if pain is not being treated sufficiently."

Joranson acknowledges the need for diversion control; however, he also stresses the importance of not restricting legitimate patients' access to drugs such as narcotics for pain. "Reluctance to prescribe opioids for intractable pain can often be attributed to physicians' perceptions that they will be investigated for violation of laws governing controlled substances. These laws and regulations amount to legal barriers to pain management. The medical use of controlled substances can provide great improvements in the quality of life for millions of people with debilitating medical conditions."

The risk of addiction to opioid drugs from cancer pain or acute pain such as post-surgical pain is indeed low; however, the risk of addiction for patients being treated for chronic, nonmalignant pain is likely to be higher, according to Russell K. Portenoy, MD, one of the nation's noted authorities on pain management and addiction. Portenoy is Director of Analgesic Studies, Pain Service, Neurology Dept., at Memorial Sloan-Kettering Cancer Center in New York City.

"There is a very large clinical experience with chronic cancer-related pain, treated in hospitals and outpatient settings, which suggests that addiction is extraordinarily rare. I've been treating cancer patients full-time for about 10 years and no more than twice have I seen an iatrogenic addiction, that is, a new addiction in a patient with no prior history of dependency," Portenoy said.

On the other hand, Portenoy's assessment of addiction among patients being treated as outpatients for chronic, nonmalignant pain suggests a different set of circumstances. "If I were to estimate, I would say that somewhere between 5% to 10% of the patients with chronic, nonmalignant pain, who are referred to pain centers, are truly addicted and have shown drug-seeking behavior. (Note that drug-craving is not the same as true addiction. Some patients are diagnosed as having "pseudo-addiction," in which their drug-seeking behaviors are driven by unrelieved pain.)

"However, some of the literature on addiction risks for chronic, nonmalignant pain sufferers suggests addiction rates as high as 17% to 30%. But I view the existing literature as totally insufficient for making a scientific determination. So, the true rate is not known, and probably varies from subpopulation to subpopulation. For example, in older people, with no prior history of substance abuse, the rate may be similar to that of cancer patients," explains Portenoy.

Understanding the area of chronic, nonmalignant pain is extremely complicated because the population is diverse. The most common, nonmalignant pain is arthritis pain; the most common pain presented to pain specialists is low back pain and headache. Other patients have medical disorders such as shingles, diabetic neuropathy, sickle cell disease and hemophilia.

"For any patient with severe chronic pain, it's best to tell them that there is a recognized pain management sub-speciality which includes specialists who are neurologists, physiologists, psychiatrists, nurses and others. The expertise of these specialists would usually go beyond that of the primary care physician."

Portenoy describes the therapies for some of these patients as "excellent" with high success rates; for other groups the therapies are "hit and miss" and the success rates are not predictable. For some patients, there's a great deal of controversy about the appropriate way to manage their pain.

One of the most important things for consumers to know today, Portenoy insists, is that pain relief is available for large numbers of patients. Widely accepted medical treatment for cancer pain shows a success rate of 70% to 90%, if a patient's physician follows a standard, accepted guideline for pain control. For acute pain, such as post-operative pain in hospital settings, the success rate for treatment is 90% to 95%.

"If patients have any concern at all that they're losing control and becoming addicted, they need to be honest about this with their physician and get an evaluation by someone who can make a proper diagnosis."

Barriers to Effective Pain Management

Problems Related to Patients:
- Reluctance to report pain
- Concern about distracting physicians from treatment of underlying disease
- Fear that pain means disease is worse
- Concern about not being a "good" patient
- Reluctance to take pain medications
- Fear of addiction or of being thought of as an addict
- Worries about unmanageable side effects
- Concern about becoming tolerant to pain medications

Problems Related to Health Care Professionals:
- Inadequate knowledge of pain management
- Poor assessment of pain
- Concern about regulation of controlled substances
- Fear of patient addiction
- Concern about side effects of analgesics
- Concern about patients becoming tolerant to analgesics

Problems Related to Health Care System:
- Low priority given to cancer pain treatment
- Inadequate reimbursement
- Restrictive regulation of controlled substances
- Problems of availability of treatment or access to treatment

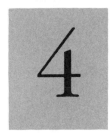

Voices of Recovery

In this chapter you'll hear from recovering addicts. Some of them underwent serious ordeals with addiction to prescription drugs that, in some cases, nearly cost them their lives. As several will explain, they were unaware that their therapeutic use of medication had escalated to abuse. And at first, most did not think they were addicted or even prone to addiction.

The individuals who tell their stories here may be referred to as "unwitting addicts" — initially, they were not drug-seekers wanting to create an altered state of consciousness. Rather, they became dependent on drugs first used to treat legitimate medical problems, both physical and emotional. As they will admit, however, the choice to eventually abuse the drugs is a choice for which they assume responsibility.

Listen carefully to their voices. Their message is clear: Recovery is possible.

As you read this chapter, remember that the majority of people who take addictive drugs do not become addicted.

Margaret, 25
Homemaker

I knew nothing about prescription drug abuse. I'd never done any sort of drugs in the past. But in 1993, I broke my arm and I was given Vicodin for pain. I ended up going through a drug ordeal for about a year and a half.

The Vicodin made me feel better — sort of a euphoria. I kept going back to the doctor and was getting prescriptions for 100 Vicodin with refills. This went on for a year and a half. No one told me the drug was addictive.

By the time my arm was getting better, I stopped taking the medication. But I would get really sick and would go to the emergency room, never equating the drugs with my migraines. So at the emergency room, I would be given Vicodin. The headache would go away. I just figured I had a migraine problem. So I continued the Vicodin for the headaches. I later realized that the headaches were from withdrawal from the drug.

Without the drug, within 24 hours I would have these really bad headaches again. I would try aspirin, but then I would start craving Vicodin. It was an addiction. It was a vicious circle.

Then, once the drug had a hold of me, I wasn't living life on life's terms. Anytime something upset me, it would be an excuse to take more medication. I could forget about my problems — much like an alcoholic would with liquor.

Because of my managed care health plan, when I went to the doctor, I rarely saw the same doctor. My addiction went undetected. When I finally did see my own doctor, he told me I had a dependency problem. I'd been taking Vicodin for a year and a half, and it was only toward the end of this time that I realized that the pills, not the headaches, were my problem.

Then, I had to go through a drug detox. It was in an out-patient program; I still had two kids to take care of. I was given other medications to help ease the discomfort. But for about seven days I stayed in my bedroom — I couldn't function at all. I couldn't sleep. I had memory problems. I was exhausted, had no energy to do anything.

For about four months, I went to personal counseling, to AA meetings and to a prescription drug abuse class. Everyday was a struggle. I had to learn how to live life all over again.

I am still afraid of relapsing. I'm horrified of ever having an injury or surgery for which I might need pain medication.

I think what really upsets me is that I was never warned once about what I was getting into in terms of taking a highly addictive drug. I didn't have a clue.

Turning Point: I was tired of being sick. Through groups and treatment I learned to make myself feel better in different ways. I started exercising a lot. I jogged and walked. I bought a stair-master. It made me feel a lot better. I started focusing on me, taking care of my emotional needs.

Advice to Others: There is light at the end of the tunnel. It may take a while, but hang in there.

Michelle, 31
Businesswoman

I had no experience with drugs — illegal or legal. I'd never even heard of most of the prescriptions I ended up taking.

After graduating from college, I started working for a large corporation. I got promoted to the position of computer system specialist. I was young and had a lot of responsibility, including oversight of 37 sales reps and their budgets. I liked it, but it was more pressure than I was used to.

In late 1987, I started getting really bad headaches and went to my doctor. At the first appointment the doctor pre-scribed Fiorinal, which I later learned was a narcotic. Within a few weeks, my headaches were continuing and so I started getting injections of Demerol. I had no idea what Demerol was. But I had a standing prescription to go into the doctor's office and have the nurse give me a shot of Demerol.

Demerol, I know now, is a Schedule II narcotic like morphine. Soon however, I was having the headaches daily,

to the point of needing to get the injections. I'd have headaches without them. But I was really getting worse and worse
headaches. My family started getting really worried about me.
We thought something was very wrong. I would wake up in
the mornings and be shaking and vomiting. I didn't realize I
was having withdrawal from the Demerol.

But my family had never been around drug users, so we
didn't know that my symptoms were actually drug withdrawal. The doctors were writing down my symptoms, but no
one seemed to suspect drug withdrawal from an opiate. Often
I got the shots from nurses, never saw a doctor. I still didn't
connect the medication with what I thought was an illness. I
was getting sicker and sicker and the medication wasn't making it better. So my family insisted that I be hospitalized for
tests. And during that hospital stay I was on an I.V. and I was
to the point by now of ordering the Demerol. I knew just
exactly what I needed in order to feel better. I'd tell the
nurse, "I need a 100 milligrams of Demerol every two to three
hours." They were doing it.

A year earlier, I'd never even heard of Demerol and now
I knew how to order it. I was asking for it...I.M. (intramuscu-
lar) or I.V., (intravenous) with Vistaril or with Phenergan.
Vistaril, a sedative, acted like a kicker and made the Demerol
last longer. Phenergan was an anti-nausea drug. I knew just
exactly what I wanted.

But within a three-day period, I'd had over a gram of
Demerol, and I had a grand mal seizure. I remember waking
up with two doctors and a nurse in the room with me. I had
blood in my mouth and all over my shirt. They told me I had
had a seizure.

So, I was never diagnosed with any illness. My problem
was Demerol. So from there, I had to go into chemical dependence recovery. My family put me in a care unit. There,
at first, I thought I was completely out of place...I was in with
addicts who were talking about "highballs" and "eightballs"
— things that I had no knowledge of. My attitude was that I
just needed to get my life back on track and be done with
doctors and drugs, but that was not the case. My doctor in

the care unit said I was the worst case of detox he'd seen from legal or illegal drugs. I was in detox seven days longer than some of the heroin addicts.

My denial was really high, because I didn't think I was truly an addict. I just thought my other doctors put me on too much medication. But I had to finally say I'm responsible for my recovery today and regardless of how I got here, I'm here. Being angry didn't really help me.

Demerol is like heroin. It's very hard to stop taking. I did finish my in-patient treatment and then started going to support groups. But I still felt out of place; I didn't think these meetings were what I needed. But a lot of prescription addicts feel out of place in 12-step meetings. Even in Narcotics Anonymous they were talking about illegal drugs and at AA meetings they were talking about alcohol, so I had a hard time fitting in. That just fed my denial — I could say none of this fits for me. I heard only the differences, not the similarities.

So I went back to work, against my doctor's advice. He told me, "Your problem is no longer headaches, your problem is about surviving. People die from this." He really wanted me to have more recovery.

But I went back to work and went out one night with friends and had a few drinks. I had never had a drinking problem so I didn't think there was any danger. But within hours of taking a couple of drinks, my craving for Demerol was back. That's how quickly it happened. I relapsed.

I felt really hopeless then. In AA you hear people talking about hitting the "bottom bottom" — when you feel like you can't live with the drugs but you can't live without them. I hated the way I was living. I opted to keep taking the drugs and to make myself be happy. I went to the Caribbean, and tried to tell myself I was okay. But it didn't take me long to end up feeling really hopeless. I knew I couldn't go on that way.

So then, I was hospitalized two or three times in psych wards; my family intervened — they wanted to help. Yet, I was angry and yelling at them. It seemed like everything that was important to me in life, everything that I cared about...I now didn't care about any of it.

The only thing that mattered was not feeling sick from the drugs...but at the same time wanting them so I could feel normal. That was all that mattered. I was angry and bitter about everything.

Turning Point: In September of '88, I took two bottles of pills — a suicide attempt. I woke up in a medical center. And maybe it was grace from above, but somehow when I woke up I felt like maybe I could get help. I remembered meeting people in support groups who, like me, had been in trouble with prescription drugs. I had a bit of hope. I thought I could return to the 12-step groups for help. I started back to AA meetings and Narcotics Anonymous.

Advice to Others: I came to realize that I was worth getting better. And every single person in that situation is. I held onto that. I found help in 12-step meetings. I found help in dealing with all my resentments about what had happened to me. I had a lot of guilt and shame, too. The support groups helped me find a way to deal with that and learn to take better care of myself. I had a supportive family, but still I had to do the work. They couldn't do it for me. I suggest reaching out to people. Learn to trust others.

Justin, 37
Attorney

I dislocated my shoulder and broke my wrist by falling down a set of stairs in 1983. It affected the nerves that ran into my neck, head and jaw so I had intense pain. Then came my first exposure to pain medication.

After a while, I told the doctor that my medication, Codeine III was not stopping the pain. He said to take two. After a couple of months, when the pain persisted, my doctor gave me Codeine IV which was twice the strength of the IIIs. So I was getting 120 milligrams per dose, prescribed for four hours apart. For two or three years I would use the medication as needed, but was gradually using it more and more. Dependency was kicking in. My tolerance was building and I really didn't realize how much I was using it. It was a very gradual thing. It never occurred to me I had a drug problem.

Two years later, my jaw pain continued so I went to a different medical center for tests and x-rays. I was told I had a problem with my jaw and needed surgery on it. However, my insurance plan would not pay for it.

So my doctors said we could only treat the pain. I told my physician I thought I was dependent on the Codeine. I knew I had a tolerance built up and if I didn't take the medication I would feel sick. I was afraid that I was becoming dependent. My doctor said it's not unusual to need ongoing medication for pain management...so I was sent to a special department for pain management. There, I was given Vicodin, which was more potent than what I was taking.

Within a couple weeks, I was really needing the drug. Every time I went back to see my doctor I would tell him I needed more pills. So I would get more. Then, I was switched to Percocet and would get occasional shots of Demerol or morphine suppositories. I also had muscle relaxants and tranquilizers.

With the opiate drugs, you build a tolerance, so others don't readily notice you're on a drug. You just need it to keep you from getting sick. However, I now realize my behavior was changing; I wasn't dealing with life normally. I would be jubilant sometimes, deeply depressed other times. My motivation to do things was affected. I managed to adjust my dosages so I could function at work, but I did call in sick a lot. I was having problems in my marriage — we eventually got divorced. I had no idea my problems were related to drug use. I just thought I was suffering from depression.

In 1986, I overdosed. I'd had a shot of Demerol, came home took some tranquilizers, went to sleep and then would wake up and take some more tranquilizers. I kept doing this, never really aware of how many pills I was taking. It's quite common, once your judgement is impaired, to not realize how many more pills you're taking.

Finally, I went to take some more and realized the bottle of 100 was nearly empty. I got really scared. I knew I was not feeling right. I called 911. When the ambulance got there, I was delirious. I ended up in the intensive care unit and almost died.

Once I got out of the hospital, I got my prescriptions refilled and started all over again. I knew the drugs were a problem but every single day was a major effort for me to try to quit. I had to have the drugs. I would get 150 milligrams of Demerol in a shot and then take Percodan.

I was feeding a real drug habit now. I tried several times to get treatment and go through detox, but then I'd still have real physical pain in my neck. Finally in 1987, I went to a specialist who performed surgery on my neck, fixed my physical problem and that ended my drug problem. I got my life together.

Looking back, I don't want to doctor bash, but it seemed the medical community didn't want to take time to explain the nature of addictive drugs. At the same time, it's not good to underprescribe drugs for pain. I've seen that problem with my mother who has legitimately needed pain medication, but couldn't get it because doctors were too cautious. I've seen both extremes. There needs to be balance.

Turning Point: It was personal realization. By the time I was taking drugs every day for three months in a row, I knew I was in trouble. I thought I could do it myself at first, but I couldn't. When I realized I couldn't stop, the more scared I became. But I was also afraid that I couldn't live without the drugs.

I became completely aware that I had a problem, but I had no idea what I could do. That made life more frightening and more depressing. I fought that for a year before I finally went for in-patient treatment. I was in for 30 days. I relapsed several times and went back into in-patient treatment seven times, ranging from five days to five weeks.

To this day, seven years later, I still go to AA meetings two or three times a week.

Advice to Others: The first thing I would say is realize you can live without the drugs. I had become 100% convinced that I could not live without them. I thought it was great that other people could recover, but I was so addicted that I thought there was no way in hell I could function without the drugs.

If someone is dependent, they may have to take a giant leap of faith and realize that they can live life without drugs. It takes some time and it's good to join a support group of people who are going through the same thing. Pair up with someone who's used a similar drug — they'll know exactly what you've gone through. Stick with these people who have been through it, and it can work for you.

Terry, 37
Nurse

I'm a nurse and ended up taking drugs on the job. This kind of thing is going on in hospitals all over. It's rampant and on the rise as far as I'm concerned. A lot of nurses need help. In one of my support groups, out of 13 of us, 7 of us were nurses. The medical profession is so intense. You're so afraid of doing something wrong. There's a lot of pressure on medical care and we have access to the drugs. Sometimes, we want to help others and do everything perfectly. That's a lot of pressure. We're only human.

My problem started in 1988, when I was a nurse on a psych ward and was injured when an enraged patient attacked me. I had a neck injury, and I was prescribed Vicodin. Eventually I had to have carpal tunnel surgery and a thumb fusion from the injury. I was on Vicodin for two years.

I loved the drug. It was wonderful. Life was easier. My husband was abusive, but when I was on the drug, whatever he did or said didn't bother me as much.

I built up a tolerance to the drug. I started taking one every three or four hours, then I'd take two. After a while, by 1991, I was taking 20 pills a day. Being a nurse, I knew this wasn't right. But no one knew I was taking so many pills. The only change in me was that my affect had become really flat. I showed no emotion.

By now, I was working in a long-term care unit and I was taking the drugs myself and signing charts as if patients were receiving them. I was the charge nurse. I had the key to the narcotics cabinet. I'd just write on a patient's chart that they'd take a certain medication, and I took it instead. The DEA requires that the drugs be recorded on a narcotics sheet, so I'd sign out the drugs to a patient. I'd write down some excuse, that the patient had a headache or back pain. Then I'd take the drugs. It was easy. This went on for a year and half. No one ever knew.

Later, I worked in a doctor's office, and in doctor's offices drug samples were available from drug salespeople. These samples were never registered, so no one knew I was taking them. Once again, I had the key to the drug cabinet. I was taking Vicodin, Xanax, Restoril, Ativan and Tylenol with Codeine.

I knew I was an addict, but thought since I was a nurse, I could stop on my own. I really tried, but I couldn't. No way. If I had stopped cold, I would have had a seizure and maybe died.

Eventually, in 1994, I was phoning pharmacies with my own prescriptions — 100 Vicodin a week. I worked for six doctors, so I would use their names, say I was calling from their office and order a script for Terry. I used five or six pharmacies. It was easy.

I was always preoccupied about getting pills, not running out. When my bottle would be less than half full I'd start to panic. I kept track on my watch — was it time to take a pill?

The end came when I got busted at work. One of the doctors caught on that I was calling different pharmacies. That was on a Friday. I was fired. I was so humiliated, really ashamed. I considered suicide, but having two children made me realize I couldn't do that. So I admitted I needed help. I didn't want the drugs, but my body did. I could not stop. I knew I was dying. I was anorexic. I was so thin I couldn't even sit on a chair because my bones were sticking out. I'd lost 73 pounds. I knew I was going to die. In my mind, death was the only way to be free of the addiction.

In fact, when you're that addicted, the cells in your body turn to the drug as their food. You don't feel like you need regular food or anything else...just that drug. If you take the drug away, it's like starving yourself to death.

So, I called a patient from our office who I knew was in recovery. She knew exactly what I needed. By Monday, I was in drug treatment. I was 15 days in detox. The first couple of days were okay, because I was being given drugs, but then my doses were gradually reduced. It was horrible. I couldn't sleep. I would shake. Just remembering what the physical withdrawal was like would keep me from ever relapsing. I ached all over. My body screamed for the pills. Muscle cramps. Diarrhea. Vomiting.

Once I was through detox, I had to start dealing with the emotional issues that caused me to drug myself in the first place, and those issues were right there, staring me in the face. I fought it like crazy because I'd been through a lot of abuse in my life and I just didn't want to feel any of the buried pain I was going to have to face. I made it but I would not have made it without the rehab center. I wouldn't have made it at home. I would have relapsed. The first 90 days is not easy.

I was blessed with a wonderful sponsor in my support group. She told me life would get better and that I deserved it. I started to believe it even though it took me awhile because I had been treated like shit all my life. I do believe in God, and my faith helped me.

Once I got out of in-patient treatment, I was scared to death — scared I would relapse. I went to two and three meetings, both AA and Narcotics Anonymous, a day for the first 90 days. That's how I did it. AA had more people with more years of sobriety, plus the structure there was good for me. In Narcotics Anonymous, the people expressed a lot of love. I needed both. I had to reach out.

With nearly a year of recovery behind me, I can't believe how good I feel. I would have never believed I could feel so happy inside. I look forward to life. I was even hired back at the doctor's office where I was fired. I still go through rough times, but if I do, I call my sponsor and I get to a meeting. I wish everyone could have the luxury of a support system like I have. All these people will help you, but you have to reach out. You do have to make that effort. You have to be willing.

Turning Point: Getting busted at work was definitely the turning point for me.

Advice for Others: Be totally honest with everyone — your friends, your therapist, whomever. Admit that your life is screwed up and admit that you need help, that you're not perfect. I found it's really neat being "not perfect." Realizing I was just another human took the weight of the world off my shoulders. Today I have freedom and love and hope in my life. It's amazing. And it gets better everyday.

Barbara, 38
Homemaker

My addiction started as a result of an injury. I hurt my back at work, picking up a heavy box. This happened in September 1992. I had surgery on my neck and wore three different braces, and even though I eventually took off the braces, the pain would not go away.

I was given Tylenol with Codeine. I also had Darvon and Vicodin. Then, the addiction cycle kicked in. I had mood swings; I was either very high or very low. I couldn't understand what was happening.

Before long, I was taking 10 pills a day. I kept a diary and noticed that I was soon up to 12 a day, then 15. By the time I was taking 25 a day, I knew I was addicted. I was a recovering alcoholic and had been sober for five years, but I knew I was addicted.

The pills began to "talk" to me. I was taking them every 20 minutes, then every 15 minutes, every 10 minutes. When I told my doctor who had prescribed all these drugs what had happened, she dropped me as a patient. She was a neurosurgeon. She told me to get an MD.

I called some women I knew from recovery groups, telling them that the pills were in charge of me and that I was dying. I couldn't tell the difference between pain in my back and psychological pain.

I went to another doctor and he gave me 90 pills of Tylenol with Codeine. I realized I was in trouble. The doctors I was seeing didn't understand addiction.

I couldn't stop taking the pills. So, I got into a hospital treatment program and was in for 20 days. I hit bottom in the hospital. I was very sick. I was vomiting. If I drank even an ounce of water I would throw up. My lowest point was when I was lying on the bathroom floor with the dry heaves.

Turning Point: The shots I was getting in detox to stop the dry heaves really burned when I got them in the hip. After about 20 of them I literally cried at the thought of getting another one. I remember falling to the bathroom floor, begging the nurses not to give me another shot. I cried and I cried and cried. I prayed like I'd never prayed before, admitting to God that I'd been an alcoholic and was now an addict and to please help me.

Advice to Others: Talk to your pharmacist to find out if a drug is addictive. Ask how long you should take it. A pharmacist will give you a lot of information if you ask for it. It's also good to get second opinions from another doctor. Especially, if you've had alcohol or drug problems, tell your doctor right up front. The opiate drugs can hook you so quickly.

Get support through AA or Narcotics Anonymous. There's a lot of wisdom in those groups. They have a lot of knowledge about different drugs and how they can affect you.

Don, 51
Realtor

My addiction to pills started in 1982 and continued for the next 11 years. I've been in recovering for several years, but continue going to a support group. I see people going through the same kinds of experiences today.

I started with a sleeping pill called Dalmane, a benzodiazepine. I was waking up very early each morning and it was really causing fatigue. At first, I took the drug as needed. Later on I took it every night at the insistence of my doctor. He said it couldn't hurt me. It worked like magic for five or six months, then I started waking up early in the morning, couldn't sleep.

Then, over the next two weeks I became severely depressed and my short-term memory was terrible. I had anxiety. Lost my sense of taste. I couldn't figure out what my problem was. I suspected the pills, but my doctor assured me it couldn't be and sent me to a psychiatrist.

But on my own, I stopped taking the drug. I realize now, looking back, I went into a serious withdrawal. I was having terrible depression and couldn't sleep. I started seeing a series of doctors and specialists, trying to find out what was wrong.

By now, I had been off the medication for a few weeks and told my doctor I had suspected the pills were my problem. He explained that the pills had a half life of 10 days — in other words the drug would have been out of my system by then. I'd been off it for a few weeks.

So I tried anti-depressants and psychiatrists. Nothing seemed to make me any better. Then I ran into a psychiatrist who put me back on a benzodiazepine, Ativan, and two or three other drugs. I did improve dramatically within a few days. Then, I stayed on these medications for years, up until 1990.

During these years, I had taken myself off the benzos a couple of times. But a few weeks later, the depression would hit me again. The doctor, who I would only see two or three times a year, would reinforce the fact that I needed the medication. So I'd go back on it.

By 1990, my life was going downhill, my business, family life. That's when I was put on another benzo and that experience became my moment of truth. The first night I took the drug I went through the worst panic attack of my life. It was the most God-awful emotional state I've ever been in. That told me that something was terribly wrong with my medication.

I searched for a few months and by the end of 1990, I found a doctor who was an addiction specialist. I also got into a support group.

I did an outpatient detox. I was put on Klonopin and tapered off in 12 weeks. It was probably too fast, and it was really difficult. Life was awful and I was suicidal. I should have taken an anti-depressant, but by that time I was too afraid of drugs.

Now, I've been drug free for several years. I'm diabetic so I take insulin. That's all.

Turning Point: The night I had the severe panic attack. That's when I knew I had to get help, and I was determined to survive.

Advice to Others: Realize that you need help with these dependencies. You cannot do it alone. Find a knowledgeable doctor — one who understands what's going on with you and find a support group. It's real essential to talk to other people who have gone through what you're going through.

Nancy, 39
Homemaker

My drug problem escalated after back surgery in 1991. I had a herniated disk. I took Vicodin and Soma, a muscle relaxant. Looking back, I realize I abused the drugs somewhat, but gave them up when my back improved. Then, in 1993, I had a second back surgery, a fusion in which they took bone out of my pelvis and put it in my spinal column. The pain afterwards was horrifying. In the hospital, I went through morphine like water — I had a high tolerance for drugs by now.

Finally, I went home, deciding I was going to take all the Vicodin I could get. I kept getting refills and abusing the pills. I was only supposed to take one every six hours, I was taking three Vicodin and three Soma every hour or two. I needed it for back pain, but I also now realize I was taking it to deal with other problems, the stress of raising my kids and a troubled marriage. I, like most addicts, was a good liar. I would lie about back pain just to get my pills.

At one point, I went to my doctor, who had prescribed Vicodin, and asked him for help. He said my problem was repetitive and that he couldn't help me. He released me as a patient. I was really angry.

In February of 1994, I knew in my own heart I was still taking too many pills, so I decided to quit on my own. I gave up Vicodin and Soma — cold turkey. I went into a grand mal seizure and was taken by ambulance to the hospital.

Consequently, I went into treatment and into a detox program. I was there for 30 days. Once I got the drugs out of my system in the first couple of weeks, I started having energy, no more diarrhea and headaches. I was acting like a human being again.

I listened to what my therapists said about addiction, and I thought I was cured. So when I came home, I took a pill which led to a relapse, a really bad one.

In treatment, they told me that inside of me was a "sleeping tiger," and even if I quit taking drugs the tiger would keep growing so that a relapse could be worse than when I stopped the drugs the first time. I learned the hard way on that.

I'm still working on sobriety. Without it, I have nothing.

Turning Point: Realizing that I had to recover for my children. I wasn't being any kind of a mother. I was in bed all day. I was a zombie. I just wanted to be able to feel like a normal person and laugh again, and not always be thinking about how I would get my next pill.

Advice to Others: Get sobriety for yourself. You can't do it for anyone but yourself. If you're in 12-step programs, work the steps. When I first went into treatment, I didn't do it for myself, I did it so I could fix things in my home life. You've got to recover for yourself.

If you go to a support meeting, AA, Al-anon, whatever, listen to what those people are saying because it works. Get phone numbers, call someone when you feel like taking a pill or drink.

Caroline Kearney Hirshfeld,
Actress, Co-Founder Benzodiazepines Anonymous

I'm a wife, a mother and I've been an actress for 25 years, working mostly in television shows and commercials. I was addicted to Xanax and nearly lost everything.

I went to only one doctor, one pharmacist. I could get 50-100 Xanax on Monday and if I wanted 100 more on Friday I could get them.

Benzodiazepines, as central nervous system depressants, can not only cause physical damage, but can hurt your belief system. They hurt my mind and my emotional well-being.

I started taking the drug after becoming extremely claustrophobic after being caught in my room on a train, in a train accident on my way East. A psychiatrist prescribed the drugs and I took them, knowing very little about them. I take responsibility for taking the pill, but I also want doctors to take responsibility and to acknowledge that some of them have problems with misprescribing.

I was chemically dependent on Xanax for over two years. After being on the drug for nine months, my panic attacks were worse. My initial symptoms returned with a vengeance. These pills can boomerang on you. It's called a rebound effect.

I didn't know it then, but I was building up a tolerance. I began taking more and more. I was so sick from taking the drug that I couldn't drive to work. I couldn't work. I wasn't able to take care of my children. I wasn't able to be a wife to my husband. I was isolating and withdrawing.

This dependency took away my dreams and my belief in myself — things I'd worked for all my life. Looking back, I see that my therapist and psychiatrist seemed uneducated about the dangers of these drugs. They said I would have no problem getting off them. But from the shape I was in, I knew in my heart and my soul that something was terribly wrong.

I entered a treatment center in August of 1987, a shell of the woman I once was. My entire stay was 40 days.

I was in the detox, withdrawing, for 12 days. I would hallucinate, and watch my fingers and hands burn off my arms. I thought I saw people losing their heads as I sat in group therapy. I lost my ability to read. I feared I would never be able to read again. I'd lost my ability to think, to analyze, to be thoughtful, to be perceptive. I had tremors. My skin felt like it was crawling, and my brain felt like it was moving — it took years before that stopped.

And I'm not alone with these symptoms. There are many other people like me. I remember seeing people coming to the treatment center who were addicted to heroin, crack, ice, cocaine and alcohol, and they were out of the detox part in three days. They were walking down the halls, strong and in command. I would watch these people as I was crawling down the same hallway. I had lost my ability to walk.

I've been off Xanax since 1987, and I'm alive today because I'm one of the fortunate ones. I lived. I am strong today. In 1989, in Los Angeles, Dr. Ronald Gershman and I co-founded Benzodiazepines Anonymous, a 12-step group for those recovering from addiction to benzodiazepines. (See resource listing on page 158.)

Turning Point: When I knew that I was ill, yet I could not stop taking the pills.

Advice to Others: Ask your doctor questions about the drugs you're getting. It's your body. It's your brain. Be knowledgeable about your medications. Don't just put yourself out there for a doctor to take care of you. Prepare yourself — it's vital.

5 Voices of Hope

In this chapter, you'll hear from professionals, including members of the American Society of Addiction Medicine (ASAM), who have treated thousands of individuals for chemical dependency. ASAM is an international association of 3,000 physicians dedicated to improving the treatment of alcoholism and other addictions.

Sidney Schnoll, MD (ASAM)
Chairman, Division of Substance Abuse
Medical College of Virginia

Our culture today treats addicts like we treated epileptics 400 years ago — we burned them at the stake because we thought they were possessed. Now we know these people have a disease which requires specific treatment. I see people who are addicted as suffering from an illness just as one who suffers from diabetes or any other illness. Yet, many see addicts as having something morally wrong with them as if it's something they bring upon themselves.

I became interested in substance abuse about 25 years ago when I was a resident at Philadelphia General Hospital. I saw a lot of young people coming in with problems — LSD use — and no one quite knew how to take care of them, and I developed an interest in addiction.

There is no one treatment for most diseases. So, there is no one specific treatment for addiction. We're talking about roads to recovery, rather than a road to recovery. It's far more complex than that. There is not one shoe that fits all. I think one of the biggest mistakes made in the field of addiction is that people make the assumption that there's one way to recover and if you don't do it that way there's something wrong with you.

For example, not every diabetic needs insulin. And those who get it take different doses. And, diabetics have different courses of progression in their disease. The same is true for addiction. It is a chronic disease just like diabetes. We can treat it, but we cannot cure it. We can control some of the symptoms. We can make some people's lives very comfortable; other people do not do as well.

Anyone who needs help with addiction should seek out the help of someone trained in the diagnosis and assessment of the problems of addiction. Addiction is not something that most physicians are adequately prepared to treat.

Le Clair Bissell, MD (ASAM)
Addictionologist, Retired
Florida

I'm an alcoholic in recovery myself so I became interested in recovery issues during my own recovery in March 1953. Some years later I went to medical school and went on to practice addiction medicine full time, from 1968 to 1982. My writing and research since I stopped seeing patients has dealt almost exclusively with substance abuse and chemical dependency.

If someone who's battling addiction feels hopeless, I would offer them the experience of other people who have recovered, along with the understanding of what the patient is feeling emotionally at the moment. Empathy without sentimentality. Also, if they're feeling really hopeless I would make a note to myself to see how many suicide attempts there have been. I'd also want to evaluate for depression. If one has come to treatment on his own, he must have a pinch of hope that things might get better, otherwise he wouldn't be there.

When it comes to treating prescription drug addiction, there are some attitudinal differences when comparing it to alcoholism. For example, a good many individuals might think it's naughty to drink, but that it's okay to have certain sedative-hyponotic pills if the doctor has prescribed them. The truth is these drugs are in the same "family" as alcohol. But pills aren't seen as being as bad as alcohol.

And all too often, these addicts are hard for doctors to spot. They haven't had the training. If the patient comes in with a clean, white shirt and clean finger nails — not the stereotype of the drug addict who lives under a bridge — many doctors will not realize the patient is an addict. The diagnosis of addiction is often made by caste and class and is made late rather than early.

If you are an addict or alcoholic in recovery, it's very important to tell your doctor so that you aren't given addictive drugs or cough syrups with alcohol. Doctors need to take a patient's history before prescribing drugs. We need to use these drugs of addiction as little and for as short a time as possible.

Over the years, I saw many patients who were doing quite well in recovery from alcoholism, but went to a physician and were given sedatives or tranquilizers. Then the mood swings began and ultimately they began to drink again. When someone, in a case like this, takes the sedation and then a couple of drinks they become very relaxed. But in a matter of a few hours, they're going to be more tense than when they started. That's when they're in the rebound. They get a down and then an up, a down and then an up. Now, if you're an alcoholic, you already have a body that knows perfectly well what you can do when those up periods feel too uncomfortable — you use more chemicals.

Now, I'm not saying anything whatsoever about the minor use of tranquilizers by people who are not addicts. There's quite a body of information that says these drugs are pretty safe for the occasional user, but for those who have already had problems with alcohol or other drugs it's a bad idea to start playing with other mood-changing drugs.

I always give this word of warning about drugs of addiction: Whenever you take a drug and that really changes the way you feel — makes you feel really good — be careful. It may be something you should not have.

Let me stress, that there are untold thousands who can use drugs wisely. But as a doctor in addiction medicine, I've seen only the casualties on the battlefield over the years. I never saw the patients who took only a few pills and used them wisely. What I saw were people who got into bad trouble and then came to me for help. I would also say to those recovering from prescription drug addiction, to be patient. It may be a while before they feel a lot better. I saw this especially with benzodiazepines. For example, someone could be clean for two months and still not feel well. It's easy to get discouraged and go back to the pills. They need to hang in...it won't always be as bad.

Finally, I would share some thoughts with families. As part of my work, I also saw many family members who suffered deeply because of a loved one's addiction. When family and friends are trying to cope with an addict it's important for them to understand several things. One, the relative or friend has to realize that they did not cause the problem and they cannot, by themselves, resolve it. Even if the addict is blaming them, they must realize they're not responsible.

Equally important, the relative has got to stop making it easy for the addict to stay sick. The parent who constantly pays the fine or bails his kid out of jail is enabling. The addict does not have to face the consequences of his own behavior.

Another thing that is important for the family to know is what a doctor is going to recommend for the patient, if treatment is underway. For example, the patient might visit a doctor and then go home and lie to the family, telling them the doctor said it was okay to take a drink or a few drugs once in a while. It helps if the family knows that what's being recommended is total abstinence from alcohol and all other mood-changing drugs of addiction.

Ronald Gershman, MD (ASAM)
Co-Founder Benzodiazepines Anonymous
Los Angeles, California

I've been a psychiatrist in private practice for the past 17 years. Most of that time I've worked in the treatment of chemical dependency. I've treated about 10 thousand patients for alcohol and drug problems and have detoxed approximately 1,500 patients for benzodiazepines — a drug which has been a strong focus of mine.

When it comes to treating patients, I see two patterns. First there is essentially the drug addict who supports an addiction through the use of prescription pills. They see themselves as different from other addicts; they often think their prescribed medication is justified even though they may be manipulating and deceptive in acquiring excessive amounts of drugs.

Secondly, I see the individuals we call the "unwitting" or "iatrogenic" addicts. These patients were put on medication, especially benzodiazepines for legitimate reasons, but for an extremely long period of time. And they're addicted.

How do such addictions occur? Benzodiazepines aside for a moment, let's look at the case of opiates, commonly used to treat pain. When people take an opiate medication, the drug relieves physical pain and it also relieves emotional pain. The problem of abuse comes in using the drug to relieve emotional pain.

For most patients, if they're using the drug strictly to relieve physical pain, when the physical pain is gone, they can give up the drug. But if they're depressed or anxious or life is miserable for them then the drug use can become a problem after the physical pain is eliminated. The emotional pain is still there and they still want to treat that pain. From what I've seen, this is a pretty clear pattern, and it's not easy to tell which patients might end up seeking the drug for emotional pain once they've healed physically.

The treatment for addiction differs dramatically on the nature of the drug you're treating. For example, treatment for a benzo addiction is very, very different from treatment for an opiate such as Vicodin or Codeine.

Managing the withdrawal and keeping the patient from relapsing is the real crux of the problem. The detox for the opiates is about 7 to 10 days and can usually be done on an outpatient basis. I use about eight different medications to help the person get through the detox. Among the medications we use in stage one withdrawal is an opiate blocker which prevents an opiate from "working" if the patient relapses.

In stage two opiate withdrawal, we use anti-depressants because the depressions are quite severe and are a major cause of relapse. Then with therapy, we help the patient learn to live and manage their sober life — which is really the heart and soul of the work that needs to be done. This detox is usually quite successful if the patient is highly motivated.

But the detox for the benzodiazepines is one of the hardest detoxes we do. It can take an extremely long time, generally, I figure about half of the length of time they've been addicted. This can range from six to eighteen months. In this recovery, the ongoing relentless withdrawals can be so incapacitating, it can cause total destruction to one's life — marriages break up, businesses are lost, bankruptcy, hospitalization and of course, suicide is probably the most single serious side effect.

All too often, this withdrawal pattern is not recognized by doctors. The patient has been on the drugs for a year or so and then the doctor says, "I don't think you need these anymore," and takes them off. In a few days when the patient breaks down, the doctor and patient assume the "old psychiatric problem" is returning. The patient is hospitalized and put on drugs. This cycle can prevent getting to the root of the dependency problem.

If benzodiazepines are used inappropriately and the patient becomes addicted, the patient builds tolerance and the drugs stop working. In fact, over a long period of time, their usage can worsen the condition they were being used to treat. What happens is, the levels of the drug in the blood drops between doses, which quickly brings on withdrawal symptoms that tend to exacerbate things. So the drug is losing its effectiveness while the withdrawal is making symptoms three or four times worse than they were before.

I believe benzodiazepines are appropriate for short-term management of acute anxiety or panic attack. Short term use meaning generally two weeks to six weeks — the absolute maximum.

David Mee-Lee, MD (ASAM)
Castle Medical Center
Honolulu, Hawaii

There is some disagreement in the medical community about the use of benzodiazepines. Although some say the benzodiazepines are over-used, some would say the opposite, that they're being underutilized out of doctors' concerns that patients will become addicted.

Opinions vary, even by country. Britain has been very strict about limiting use of benzodiazepines to shorter term use. In the United States, the fear of abuse has been over-blown and patients are being robbed of adequate use because of fear of addiction.

My view is that these drugs are like alcohol, in that, not everyone is going to use them inappropriately. I think long-term use can be acceptable as long as the risks and benefits are weighed cautiously and careful assessment of the patient is done to make sure those at high risk for addiction are screened out.

Even if a patient is not at high risk for addiction, the physician should always periodically reassess the use of any medication to see if the patient still needs it. I don't believe drugs should be prescribed blindly just because the patient is not becoming addicted. There are other ways to cope.

Of course, anyone taking even therapeutic doses of ben-zodiazepines for a period of time will become tolerant of the drug and would have be gradually withdrawn from it. To quit abruptly would cause withdrawal. But not everyone would have to be detoxed on an in-patient basis.

The people who often get in trouble are those who would have escalated their use of the drug; they would be at high dosages and often be in a poor recovery environment, have lack of support and have poor impulse control in terms of relapse. Most people will do better if they have motivation to come off the drug and have more resources, both personally and environmentally, to help them deal with impulsive use.

Prescription drug addiction is a very real part of the addiction population we serve. I see a lot of poly-drug use, or use of various drugs in combination — some legal, some illegal.

We need to understand a couple of basics about addic-tion, in general. One, that addiction is something that affects not only the person using, but those around — family and friends. There are very few families who aren't affected by addiction in some way. And also, the one who has the problem needs to acknowledge that there is a problem. Fam-ily members and others can be helpful by confronting and not rescuing the person.

The patients who obtain pharmaceuticals through legal means, but yet escalate dosages and abuse the drugs, often have trouble admitting to their problem. They tend to say they were just doing what their doctors told them. They don't see themselves as addicts. We try to help these patients see that their drug use has been negatively affecting their lives.

Some of these patients come to treatment once their doc-tor has judged they've become addicted and has stopped prescribing. The patients are sometimes left not knowing what to do if they're not guided into treatment.

What goes into successful recovery? Anyone can succeed. The degree of difficulty depends on how much damage has already been done. Has the patient lost jobs, family and physical health? The more one has lost, the harder recovery

Table 7. Stages of Chemical Dependence

Stage	Description
Abstinence	Person has not begun to use drug, but attitudes are developing
Non-problem use	No negative consequences of use
High-risk use	Use is frequent, heavy, or usage patterns are dangerous
Problem use (or abuse)	First negative consequences arise from usage patterns
Chemical dependence: Early stage	Reversible, less serious negative consequences of threats do not motivate corrective adjustment of usage patterns
Chemical dependence: Middle Stage	Irreversible negative consequences of use do not motivate significant corrective adjustment of usage patterns
Chemical dependence: Late stage	Multiple, serious irreversible negative consequences have failed to motivate corrective adjustment of usage patterns

Source: From "Finding Substance Abusers," by M.R. Liepman, *et al.*, 1984. *Family Medicine Curriculum Guide to Substance Abuse.* (Society for Teachers of Family Medicine, Kansas City, Mo.) Copyright 1984. Reprinted by permission.

might be for them, compared to someone who has not yet experienced many losses because of the addiction (See Table 7).

Then, in recovery, it's like any other chronic illness. You have to keep monitoring it to make sure you're taking care of yourself. For people with addictions it means continuing in some kind of recovery program. That doesn't mean going to support groups daily for the rest of your life, but rather continuing to be vigilant about relapse and using support groups or other methods to stay aware.

Some people can recover on their own. They come to the awareness that they have a problem and decide to do something about it. Not everyone goes through treatment. Many people can do something about it themselves; others need help.

And, in the scenario in which the addict won't get into recovery, his or her family can still recover. They can learn to stop playing into the addict's agenda and learn to stop passing the problem on down through generation after generation.

In short, people with the chemical dependencies must first remember that they have an illness. Second, that they're at risk for relapse and third, that they need ways to cope with stress or problems if they're heading toward relapse. It's that way with any illness.

Addiction is a chronic illness, not a moral problem. It needs treatment, not judgment.

Patrick Dalton, Certified Addiction Counselor
Addiction Institute
Costa Mesa, California

On a scale of 1 to 10, how serious is prescription drug abuse in the United States? I would say a 10.

The individuals we see are out-patients. Many are addicted to prescription drugs. We insist that they divulge all information about the drugs they are taking in order for us to treat them effectively. Often, they're getting drugs from doctors who aren't aware of addiction issues. The doctor might be trying to eliminate a patient's pain, but not understand potential addiction problems. If the patient is prone to addiction, this can be like feeding gasoline to a fire.

Those dependent on prescription drugs have a mindset different from that of alcoholics. Most of the people I've treat are very resistant to letting go of their drugs. They can partially justify it because they've gotten their drugs legitimately, from a doctor. They don't have the stigma of being a user of street drugs. This causes a high degree of relapse.

In addition to this denial, those who are prescription-drug dependent have a real fear of not being able to cope without their drugs. They are very "med-seeking," always wanting a pill to fix them.

Some people don't realize they are prone to addiction, and they get hooked on a legal drug. They may not realize it until they start having negative consequences in their lives. When you use a chemical of any kind once it's brought negative consequences to your life, you're crossing the line into addiction. Anyone who is aware of his addictive tendencies, should always tell a treating physician.

Who's to blame for this national drug problem? Given all the drugs we have available...maybe it's science.

We're still learning. Look how long Alcoholics Anonymous has been around, since 1935, and just recently we're seeing a possible hereditary factor in alcoholism.

Shiela Blume, MD (ASAM)
South Oaks Hospital
Amityville, New York

There are many kinds of prescription drugs, but when it comes to those involved in addictions, we're talking about sedative-hypnotics, stimulants or the opiates and their derivatives which are, perhaps, causing the most problems today. These are such drugs as Darvon, Vicodin and the analgesics which have Codeine in them.

Not everyone who uses them gets addicted, but anyone who does take them should be warned of their addictive potential. In my experience, those who become addicted to these drugs fall into several categories. The most common is the person who is an alcoholic but doesn't know it — the alcoholism hasn't been diagnosed yet and the person is being seen for associated symptoms such as insomnia, tension, difficulty concentrating. Then, another drug is prescribed and the patient becomes addicted.

Even sadder, is the patient who has recovered from alcoholism or other addictions, but does not understand about the addiction potential of other drugs and becomes addicted to them. These can be people who may have recovered from earlier addictions on their own, without treatment or self-help groups. Many, many people do this. However, if they haven't been in a treatment program, they may not have been educated about other mood-altering drugs. This knowledge could have saved many self-recovering people from additional trouble.

I recall the case of one man, a recovering alcoholic, who had separated his shoulder. Because he had stopped using alcohol on his own, he really didn't see himself as an alcoholic. So, when he was given Tylenol with Codeine for pain, he got hooked on it and, in the end, it almost killed him.

All recovering addicts need to tell any doctor, including dentists, that they should not take habit-forming drugs. If a doctor tells a recovering patient that the drugs won't cause dependency problems, but the patient still isn't sure, he should make another check with the pharmacist about any such dangers with the drug.

Another category of people who are susceptible to dependence are those in a lot of emotional distress or agitation. Once prescribed a sedative or tranquilizer, they can become dependent. For people who have not been drug-dependent before, the first symptom of dependence is that the drug becomes very precious to them. They are very solicitous to have it with them at all times, to have the prescription refilled well in advance so they won't run out. They think it's the most wonderful thing in the world — it's really helped them.

Then when they hit a point where something bothers them emotionally, they take a little extra of the drug and that feels good. Then, they begin to increase the dose. At this point, they may get wary, and decide not to tell their doctor about how they're using the drug. They fear their doctor won't approve and will stop prescribing. They begin to justify their use of the drug through denial or rationalization. They might start to manipulate the doctor, saying they lost a prescription or they're going on a trip and need extra pills. This works for only a short time so then they'll have to switch to another doctor. They may have five or six doctors they can reliably go to. They know exactly what drug they want when they schedule the appointment. There is a point when abuse becomes addiction. Abuse refers to dangerous use...like taking a drug and driving when you should not be driving while under the influence of the drug. And often people can stop at abuse, but if they don't they move on to dependence. At this point, they are preoccupied with the drug, always having it. Making sure they never run out. Taking extra doses. Trying to cut down and not being able to do so.

My message of hope is that prescription drug addiction is a treatable disease. Sometimes it's harder to do an intervention with prescription drugs than with alcohol or illegal drugs; patients often believes they really don't need it. But treatment can work. Recovery is very possible.

David Gastfriend, MD (ASAM)
Massachusetts General Hospital
Boston, Massachusetts

I would say about 15% of our practice involves prescription drug dependence. We see a range of patients.

At one end of the range, is the patient who has been prescribed a drug from the Valium family, like Xanax, for treatment of panic disorder. Initially they got relief from the drug, but then needed increased doses to achieve their state of comfort. Then, they simply have difficulty coming off the medication, even though they want to discontinue it. This is a case of physiological dependence, not an addiction, and it's very common with these medications even when they are used correctly and safely. Treatment is a matter of tapering the doses, educating the patient about what to expect and teaching the patient to use behavioral techniques to cope with modest withdrawal symptoms. This is the most common problem we see.

At the extreme end of the range are those who are fully dependent on either alcohol, cocaine or narcotics who are compulsively seeking to get high. They will use prescription drugs in combination with illegal drugs. Or when they can't get heroin, they'll substitute with prescription opiates or benzodiazepines. They are truly addicted, manipulative and compelled by their disease to gain the system. Often they feign illness to multiple doctors. These patients make up a smaller element of the overall problem, but it's a very costly problem in terms of death, emergency room visits, thefts, auto accidents, firearm accidents, drug trading and the like.

The mid-range of patients that I see are those who have been prescribed medications, and who have psychological problems, although these problems initially may not have been apparent. Problems such as dependency on others, impulsiveness under stress and paranoia. For these patients, certain drugs can create physiological and psychological dependence. This begins the cycle of addiction, which is compulsive use which results in an urge to maintain use of the substance at high personal costs.

We know there are individuals who are highly vulnerable to becoming alcoholic for genetic reasons. We don't have reliable research information on genetic vulnerability to addiction to anxiety medication and prescription analgesics or narcotics. But, there is work developing that infers that the same possibility for addiction exists. Many drugs have the same physiological effects as alcohol.

Patients in this category are often referred to us addiction specialists, once their doctors realize they're being manipulated into prescribing excessive doses; the doctor may not want to cut off the patient completely from the drug, and will call for a consultation with an addiction specialist.

There are warning signs that indicate prescription drug use is becoming problematic. Addiction problems could be arising when:

1. You start to feel that the drug, at the same dose, isn't working as well as it used to.
2. You feel the drug wearing off before it's time to take the next dose.

3. You experience more than symptom relief as the drug takes effect; there is some degree of excitement or high. This indicates the dose may be excessive or that the medication may work too rapidly for safe, long-term use.

4. You feel subdued or lethargic within a few hours of taking the medication. This may be an another indication that the dose is excessive.

5. You're irritable and have problems sleeping. Here, the medication may be too-short acting and maybe produces mild withdrawal over the course of the sleep cycle.

6. You feel that you can only perform certain tasks or engage in certain activities — like driving through traffic or socializing at a party — with the benefit of the medication. This feeling increases with time.

If you note any of these warning signs, you should speak to your physician about it. Ask the doctor if a consultation would be a good idea. Also, review your past history and your family history for substance use. Look for potential warning signs — parent's, grandparent's or sibling's response to similar medications or substances like alcohol.

If a patient has run into problems with a drug, we expect them to take some responsibility for their behavior and ask for help. Many are afraid to ask questions for fear they'll be cut off from the drug and they'll suffer. But in order to reasonably and ethically prescribe some of these medications, the physician counts on the patient to be a partner in fostering good health.

Jeff Baldwin, PharmD
Associate Professor of Pharmacy
University of Nebraska College of Pharmacy
Omaha, Nebraska

It's important to recognize that there's not a specific level of drug or alcohol use that determines when you're addicted. For example, I've seen a woman who was alcoholic on one beer a day, and I've seen a man who was alcoholic on a case of beer a day. The better definition of addiction is "continuing to use a substance once it brings negative consequences to your life."

Once we do have an addiction, I believe one of the most important things for recovering is faithfully going to meetings, 12-step or support groups. And, recovering people who first go to 12-step groups also should understand that they may need to be on some medications during their recovery; however, many attending those meetings mean well, but will say that if you're taking any drug that has mood-altering properties, you are not "clean." This is wrong. They're off base.

In fact, some 40% of alcoholics and addicts have a dual diagnosis, meaning they have other clinically apparent psychiatric illnesses that require medication. Manic depression, for example. Other people might need anti-depressants — the only way they can get well is when the demons quit hollering around in their heads and they're not depressed all the time.

Further, it may help those who have gotten off addictive drugs to understand that, at some point in their lives, they may have to take controlled substance drugs for medical reasons — like for pain after surgery. This is not a death sentence, but needs to be treated carefully by the health professional and the patient. The patient should be given no more of the drug than is absolutely necessary. And, probably the best thing to do is to treat the experience as if it were a relapse. Assume that the patient will lose control of the decision to use or not to use the drug excessively. In other words, it's a controlled relapse. It's not truly drug-seeking behavior.

Also, if you have a dependency, find a physician who understands addiction. You also need a pharmacist who understands addiction so, for example, if you need an over-the-counter cold preparation, the pharmacists can help you choose the ones safer for you.

We need to remember, too, that once someone has been addicted, they're not immune from becoming addicted to other substances...such as alcohol, even if they've never been alcoholic. That's often tough for people to accept — that alcohol is risky. But once they've been addicted to a mood-altering substance and they have the brain chemistry that predisposes them to dependency, they're at risk.

The use of alcohol can lead to drug relapse. Alcohol can lower their inhibitions and they decide to "use" again. It's also common to switch addictions — from pills to alcohol or vice versa.

Recovering individuals also should know about relapse counseling. This involves teaching the recovering person to recognize the early warning signals for impending relapse. Relapse is not just picking up a pill all of a sudden and taking it. Relapse is a long path of events; individuals can usually identify the sorts of things that lead them in a downhill spiral toward relapse.

For example, someone might start feeling anxious and start acting out — sexually, or spending money or being nasty with people. These may be warning signs that they need to get back to support meetings and talk to people. They're starting to isolate, which is a set up for relapse.

Terence T. Gorski, MA
Recovery and Relapse Prevention Specialist
Homewood, Illinois

As long as we've had treatment, we've had relapse. We've always had strategies for relapse prevention, but normally the strategy was simply to do the same treatment program that already may have not worked very well.

There is no such thing as a hopeless addict. There are only those who haven't found out about relapse prevention techniques. Basically, relapse prevention therapy is based upon the premise that there are observable warning signs that occur before a person returns to alcohol or drug use.

The easiest way to explain it is to look at a model: the first thing that happens is there is some stress or change that occurs in a person's life. The change or stress then triggers a change in thinking — one begins using old, addictive thinking strategies which then triggers a change in feeling. The person begins feeling painful, distressful, unmanageable feelings. This produces a change in behavior in which the person begins using self-defeating or compulsive behaviors to cope with the feelings. This brings about a change in situations; that is, the person starts hanging around people, places and things where the self-destructive behavior is tolerated.

What should you do when you start recognizing these warning signals? The first thing is identify your own unique pattern of relapse signs. Every recovering person has relapse warning signs, and they are like fingerprints — everybody has them, but each person's are different. You should write down your own personal list of relapse warning signs and describe how they move you from stable recovery back toward alcohol or drug use. You also need feedback from outside sources, because the recovering person is locked in a delusional system and can't always see what's really going on in life.

One of the most important things I've learned about recovery is that if you've been dependent on drugs or alcohol, you cannot safely use these substances. The goal needs to be to learn how to live a drug-free life. To do this, you have to learn how to think clearly, logically and rationally in a sober state. You need to learn how to recognize, label and communicate your feelings and emotions in a sober state. And you have to learn how to self-regulate your behavior as a sober person. You must re-adjust from an addiction-centered social life to a sobriety-centered social life.

Addiction has several facets — biological, psychological and social. People can become dependent on any one of these levels or all three simultaneously. Biological dependency means a tissue dependency on a drug which then creates tolerance and withdrawal. With psychological dependence, a person has come to rely on alcohol and drugs in order to manage their thinking, feeling and behaviors. Without these substances, they can't think clearly or deal with feelings. They can't self-regulate their behaviors. Social dependency means that a person has come to rely on alcohol or drugs to act as a social lubricant or social facilitator; without these, they cannot maintain satisfactory relationships with others.

There was a fascinating research study by Dr. Stanley Gitlow in the 1960s with heroin addicts and non-heroin addicts in the V.A. system. It shows there's more to addiction than just the biological addiction.

Gitlow invited heroin addicts who were "clean and sober" in treatment to be in an experiment where they would be re-addicted to heroin in a controlled setting. Gitlow took other patients who were never addicted to heroin but who agreed to become addicted to it.

Then, he had all of them stop using heroin, cold turkey. Then, he offered them free access to heroin if they desired. Ninety percent of the previously non-addicted people, even though they had become tissue tolerant or biologically addicted, did not want to start again. One hundred percent of the addicts did want to start again. The point is, once they were addicted, they needed the drug to function. So there's more to addiction than the physiology of it.

To offer hope, remember there are many, many avenues for getting help. It starts out with the most readily available form of help which is the 12-step groups, A.A. or others. The help goes on through a continuum of out-patient and in-patient services.

It's very important to realize that you cannot do it alone. If you take 100 people and have them all try to stop using a substance on their own, about 93 of them will return to use. You need social support and need to learn skills to deal with life sober. Learning how to be sober is a skill-training experience. You have to learn to depend on something besides alcohol or drugs to deal with your thoughts, feelings, relationships and behaviors.

PART
TWO

How Prescription
Drugs Are Diverted

6 Why Physicians Misprescribe

It's estimated that between 80% and 90% of all pharmaceutical drug diversions occurs in doctors' offices, at pharmacy counters or in hospitals. Doctor-shoppers and pharmacy-shoppers constitute the greatest portion of prescription drug diversion. Many are acquiring drugs to self-medicate; others may be reselling the drugs.

Although health professionals have virtually no control over a medication after the point of sale, the American Medical Association (AMA) has adopted a Four-D physician classification to explain why physicians might misprescribe. The four categories are: duped, dated, disabled and dishonest (See Table 8).

Duped or deceived

Here, the physician is most vulnerable and the greatest amount of diversion occurs. The physician, failing to detect deception, is manipulated into prescribing drugs for a dishonest patient. It is the patient who has failed to meet his or her responsibility in the patient-physician relationship (See Table 9). The scams used by the deceiving patient range from the simple to the elaborate. Given the right circumstances, any physician could be deceived for a period of time.

Table 8. Physician and Patient Contribution in the AMA Categories of Misprescribing Physicians

AMA Category	Physician's Contribution	Patient's Contribution
Dated	Fails to keep current with prescribing practices or knowledge about current drug abuse patterns	. . . .
Disabled	Fails to exercise optimal judgment because of impairment	. . . .
Dishonest	Subverts medical practice for personal gain.	Uses doctor as drug dealer, not for medical care.
Duped	Fails to detect deception. Allows himself or herself to be manipulated into prescribing at variance with accepted medical practices.	Falsifies or withholds information.

Dated

The dated doctor fails to keep current with prescribing practices or knowledge about current drug abuse patterns. A physician might misprescribe psychoactive drugs because the data on which that prescription is based are obsolete.

A number of doctors acknowledge that many medical schools do not adequately teach how to prescribe controlled substances. For many years, the view that drug and alcohol abuse were moral problems has resulted in the omission of these subjects from medical school coursework. Other physicians claim that too many of their colleagues are unprepared to diagnose and treat addiction.

Table 9. Physician and Patient Responsibilities for Preventing Drug Abuse

Responsibilities of Physician	Responsibilities of Patient
To have patient's well-being as primary concern.	To seek medical attention for conditions which patients believes a physician can cure or ameliorate.
To formulate working diagnosis of the patient's problems based on the patient's history and by examination of the patient.	To be truthful in relating historical information and to cooperate with the physical examination.
To order appropriate lab tests (or consultations with specialist) to clarify a diagnosis.	To obtain the lab tests or consultations requested by the physician.
To prescribe appropriate therapy. (This assumes the physician is acting within his/her scope of expertise.)	To comply with the physician's instructions. (This includes taking medications as prescribed.)
To monitor the effect of treatment, including the side effects of toxicity of any drugs prescribed.	To report symptoms accurately.
To continue follow-up until the condition is relieved or the patient's care is assumed by another physician.	To follow through with appointments until discharged by the physician.

"Doctors need education on addictions and the potential dangers of addictive drugs," states Ronald Gershman, MD, Los Angeles. "Addiction has not been a part of traditional medical training. And, many physicians are not interested in addiction. For example, a cardiovascular surgeon doesn't have the time or the interest or perceived need to learn about benzodiazepines and their addictive properties.

"Roughly 70% of physicians specialize in one area, yet they can prescribe all medications. It's dangerous to rely on the idea that we can depend on physician competence and their capacity to self-educate. If we do this, millions of people can be harmed. The evidence speaks for itself. Millions of people have gone through these nightmares with iatrogenic addiction.

"With computers and molecular modeling, technology is evolving extremely rapidly in terms of how we manufacture and create drugs. It can be difficult to keep pace with all the new data. Physicians easily understand the traditional compounds — opiates, barbiturates, but these newer drugs have been replaced by compounds with enormously greater complexity. The benzodiazepines are an example. We have never appropriately appreciated the really severe potential or addictive potential of these drugs and their potential for harm.

"The mandate, I think, is to protect the welfare of the average consumer. I refer to this consumer as 'innocent,' compared to the true addict who bases their use and abuse on prescription drugs; this is a much smaller element. The misuse of these drugs is a great danger."

Dishonest

According to AMA, only 1%, 5,000 to 7,000, of the nation's doctors fall into the "dishonest" category. These physicians, or so-called "script docs," are those who use their medical licenses to deal drugs. Even though only a very small percentage of health professionals are considered dishonest, this group of professionals has been known to illegally prescribe vast quantities of drugs. In Tennessee, for example, one DEA survey showed that of the 10,000 health professionals eligible to order narcotics, 38 had ordered half of all narcotics shipped to Tennessee; 3 doctors had ordered 22% of the state's narcotics.

As one California Bureau of Narcotic Enforcement agent explained, "We talk to addicts who are informants, and they tell us which doctors they go to. The informants say, 'All you have to do is give the doctor some phoney excuse. He just needs something to write down [as an illness], and he'll charge you $150 for it. You probably spend about five minutes there.'"

Disabled (Impaired)

The disabled physician misprescribes because of his or her own impairment — mental illness or misuse of self-prescribed psychotropic medications. Several studies show that health professionals have a higher prevalence of substance abuse than the general population. This trend is due, in part, to physicians' access to controlled substances. Narcotics rank second as the chemical substances misused by health professionals; alcohol ranks first.

Another study estimates that two percent of the nation's physicians are chemically impaired each year. The same research points out that 8% of physicians are chemically dependent at some point in their lifetimes.

"If you're going to have a medical license, you should be drug tested," insists Robert L. DuPont, MD. "I don't understand a society that says we will test bus drivers, but we won't test surgeons."

There are, perhaps, "gray areas" in the AMA's 4-D classifications. Some doctors describe the "GOMER" syndrome — "Get out of my emergency room" scenario in which a tired, exasperated doctor may write a prescription in order to be rid of a demanding patient.

Other doctors have described the dilemma that often occurs with patients whose families they've treated for years. One retired physician, an internist in family practice in the Midwest, cites an example of a tough judgment call. "Let's say you get a midnight call from the adult daughter of one of your elderly patients; the daughter is beside herself — her mother is not sleeping, is agitated and anxious. Do I as the physician take the hard-nosed approach and say tranquilizers may not be appropriate for this elderly patient — the drugs could be abused? Or do I do the compassionate thing and try to help this patient and family who's suffering? If I do, some might call this inappropriate prescribing. But we family physicians know what it's like to get these calls at midnight, on weekends or holidays. These issues are not always black and white."

7 How Drugs are Diverted from Pharmacies

Nearly 5 million prescriptions are filled daily in the nation's 112,000 community pharmacies. The professionals behind the counters, the pharmacists, are the last barrier between the drug abuser and his or her drug of choice. The average pharmacist rejects one to two prescriptions per week; however, untold numbers of prescriptions are dispensed as the result of fraud by customers. Many experienced drug seekers believe that health professionals, due to their training and professionalism, can be easily exploited.

Techniques for Diverting Drugs from Pharmacies*

- Forging prescriptions
- Passing fraudulently obtained prescriptions (patient feigned illness or doctor was dishonest)
- Posing as physician, in person or by telephone
- Theft, robbery or elaborate scams

---

*Brian Goldman, MD *Unmasking the Illicit Drug Seeker*, ed. William P. Egherman, MD (Hagerman, Idaho: CME-TV, Inc., 1993), 2.

Prescription forgery is the most popular diversion technique because:

- it can be lucrative
- it's perceived by offenders as victimless
- chances of arrest are often minimal
- if apprehended, penalties are often minimal
- 85% of all forged prescriptions are filled

The range of customers visiting pharmacies are:

- Appropriate users of controlled drugs
- Inappropriate users of controlled drugs
- Chemically dependent patients
- Entrepreneurial patients — con-artists, seeking drugs for resale
- "Professional" patients — individuals appearing to have legitimate ailments (scars, amputations) who are "recruited" by scammers to obtain prescriptions from physicians

How might pharmacies better protect themselves from diversion? According to Gary Holt, PhD, the role of pharmacy needs to shift from that of providing pharmaceutical "services" to that of pharmaceutical "care." Meantime, Rob Waspe, a former drug store chain attorney for 13 years, explains the economics behind today's focus on high-volume sales.

Gary Holt, PhD
Professor of Pharmacy, Northeast Louisiana University
Monroe, Louisiana

Pharmacies have been moving more toward the McDonalds fast-food approach to dispensing medicine in the past two decades. The advisory role of pharmacists has not developed like it could have, although efforts are now being made to enhance the professional role of pharmacists.

Pharmacy has not been very successful at balancing the retail component of their stores from the professional component. On one side of the store, we sell drugs, one of the most highly-controlled products in the country, and on the other side of the store we sell barbecue grills and Halloween masks. Pharmacies are pressured, either from internal pressure to make profits, or by the consumer, to treat drugs as if they are like other products in the store.

Pharmacists need to be able to interact with customers more, but studies show that in many heavily worked environments, pharmacists are pressured to dispense more, not interact with patients. Too often, the pharmacists become technicians, not professionals available to counsel patients about medications. I once had a supervisor tell me, "We pay you to type labels, not visit with customers."

Many of these work scenarios are daunting. National studies that show once you start filling more than 10 scripts an hour, error rates increase. A lot of pharmacists are concerned about this, especially once they have to start doing levels of 200-400 scripts a day. In fact, I worked for a pharmacy in Oklahoma City, where we filled 1,500 scripts a day. It wasn't a professional environment. It was nothing but a sweat shop.

A pharmacist can learn a lot from the written script itself, but given the time to do so, a traincd pharmacist can discover a lot about patients by talking to them. But if pharmacists are hogtied behind the counter filling scripts, forged prescriptions can fly past them all day long and they'll never be able to catch it. Some of the forged prescription writers are clever, and if you don't have time to examine these scripts as they flash under your nose, they can slip by much more easily.

Even when forgeries are spotted, many pharmacists are reluctant to report them to police. The problem involves a flaw in our justice system. I'll tell you why, based on my own experience.

I was working in a pharmacy several years ago when a guy handed me a suspicious script. The guy was wearing black, high-topped boots, blue-jeans with a tow-chain for a belt, black leather jacket, long hair and huge moustache.

I phoned the doctor and confirmed that the script was bogus. So I called the police. They were right across the street, so by the time I hung up the phone, the officers were walking in the door. They arrested this man as he stood in front of the pharmacy counter. Then began the games of the legal system.

A few weeks later, I was instructed to appear in court. Failure to appear is a crime itself. So, of course, I show up in court. I had waited for three to four hours before I was told the case was postponed. So I went home. It was an inconvenience — I'd lost a half-day at work.

Two weeks later, I went back to court. Again, I waited hours. Again, the case was postponed. The attorney for the defendant was hoping that I eventually would not show up, and since I was the witness, the case would be automatically thrown out of court. I was told this is a common practice — keep postponing the case until the witness becomes sufficiently frustrated to not appear.

We finally had the hearing about six weeks after the initial arrest. When the defendant came into the courtroom, he'd had a total makeover. He was no longer a motorcycle rogue. He was clean shaven, his hair had been cut and he wore a suit. The whole crux of the defense was, "Can you recognize him?"

Right or wrong, the issue here was not guilt or innocence, but rather court room chicanery. This was an example of our legal system being without ethics. There was only one principle: Win any way you can. Freeing guilty individuals often bears no weight on the conscience of the legal system.

In the courtroom that day, there was no question in my mind I was looking at the same guy who'd passed me the forged script. But I'd only seen him for a few minutes six weeks earlier, and I was supposed to swear it was the same guy?

When I was asked by the defendant's attorney, if the man in the suit was the guy I saw in the store, I could only say "I think it is." The attorney harassed me, pointing out 20 guys in the courtroom had moustaches...how, he asked, did I not know if one of them was the suspect?

Eventually, the guy was convicted. My story is not unique. I hear routinely from other pharmacists that they're tired of similar tactics used by the legal system. I have yet to go to a meeting of pharmacists where I don't hear stories of similar experiences. Consequently, a lot of pharmacists just don't want to report someone because of the abusive nature of the court system. The pharmacists may simply give a suspicious script back to the customer or may tell them they're out of the drug. Unfortunately, some pharmacists will fill the script...and add on an "annoyance fee."

Finally, I think a great portion of the solution lies beyond the pharmacies, the doctors, and justice system...and with us as consumers. We need to take some self-responsibility. We need to relearn how to cope with the emotional stressors of life. It's so easy to pop a pill, but a pill is not a solution. Trouble is, the pill wears off; the problem returns and you're just as stressed as before. Somehow we are going to have to rethink how we live our lives and how we handle stress. We can't continue the credo: "Reality is for people who can't handle drugs." But until we change, we are going to have people who will abuse drugs and find ways to scam the system.

As for pharmacists, their potential to improve the system of "pharacemtical care" is great. We have more pharmacists than any other health professionals in our nation's communities. And repeatedly, pharmacists are mentioned as the most-trusted professionals in Gallup polls. Their knowledge, combined with their community availability, provides untapped potential for providing important health care changes in the future.

Rob Waspe, Attorney
Former Vice President & General Counsel for Drug Store Chain

I understand pharmacy's focus on revenue. The practice of pharmacy has changed fundamentally over the years.

Twenty years ago, a pharmacist was probably filling 50 to 60 prescriptions a day. Customers paid cash and the pharmacist was making enough money to cover operating costs and show a profit. The pharmacist also had time to become involved with customers.

Today however, the profit margins have changed. First, most prescriptions are paid for by a third party — insurance. These profit margins have been in a constant downward spiral for the last 15 years. Gross profit margins for pharmacy departments have eroded 15% to 18%. What has been the result of these thin margins? Volume selling has become the name of the game.

Perhaps drug manufacturers are making record-breaking profits, but the opposite is true for pharmacies. Some pharmacies are not generating much revenue in their drug departments, but rather their revenues are coming from the sale of other items in the stores.

The pressure to sell, I'm sure, effects pharmacy owners in various ways. If a manager criticizes a pharmacist for not selling enough, the pharmacist may pay more attention to numbers than to a suspicious prescription. Conversely, some pharmacists will not do anything to jeopardize their licenses.

Despite the focus on volume selling, the base line of accepted performance by pharmacists is compliance with all legal requirements. Under the Controlled Substance Act, a pharmacist is not authorized to dispense a prescription if he or she does not believe, in good faith, that the prescription is valid.

Carmen Catizone, Executive Director
National Association of Boards of Pharmacy
Parkridge, Illinois

Are there dishonest pharmacists out there? How many pharmacists might be breaking the law? I'd say pharmacists would be below the average. If the national statistics for dishonest doctors is 1% or 2%, I'd say the percentage of dishonest pharmacists would rank no higher than those percentages.

In the United States, 191,000 pharmacists are licensed; 180,000 of these are actively practicing. In 1993, the 50 states combined reported 1,088 total disciplinary actions. To date, we've seen, on average, only six license revocations per state per year. Quite a low number. Our data base, however, does not tell us what the infraction was that brought about the disciplinary action.

As a regulatory organization, our role is to assist state boards in protecting the public's health. We watch what's happening with disciplinary actions against pharmacists across the nation. We are the central disciplinary clearing house. We consider diversion a serious issue. We develop model regulations and model laws. For example, we proposed the requirement that pharmacists counsel Medicaid patients; this was passed into federal legislation. In forty states, the offer is supposed to be made to counsel all patients. When we develop laws or rules on how to deal with diversion, we pass them on to the states and the states pass them as they see fit. Pharmacists need to take an active role in reporting diversion or suspected diversion. We know some are reluctant to report it.

8 Scams for Drugs

A woman shows up in a doctor's office, saying she's just moved to town; she tells the physician that she has chronic back pain and Vicodin is the only drug that gives her relief. The physician prescribes the drug. The woman leaves, using the drug to alter her mood. She does not have back trouble.

In another city, a young man appears in a hospital emergency room on the weekend, complaining of severe toothache. He can't see his dentist until Monday and needs a painkiller badly, he insists. The man leaves with a prescription for Tylenol with Codeine, a drug he'll use to numb emotional pain.

Other common scams by drug abusers who self-medicate include feigning such ailments as headache, back pain or kidney stone attacks. These self-diagnosing drug-seekers usually request specific medications and show no interest in confirming a diagnosis or undertaking other forms of treatment.

Untold numbers of scams are perpetrated on health professionals every day. Many scammers are planning to divert the drugs for profit. Others are acquiring drugs purely to self-medicate.

"Jeff," a businessman from Omaha, used prescription drugs to feed a habit, and became very adept at obtaining them.

Jeff, 34
Businessman

I was coming off a year's binge with cocaine. I had gone through several hundred thousand dollars' worth of coke. I lost my house, my friends, my job. I could no longer afford cocaine, so I went back to morphine and Demerol which I'd been on as a teenager after being seriously injured by a shotgun blast in a hunting accident.

In the beginning of my drug seeking, I went to doctors' offices, feigning back ailments to get prescriptions. But a lot of doctors were suspicious and I didn't get what I wanted. I could get some prescriptions but not for the heavy drugs I wanted or for the quantities I needed. I really wasn't quenching the habit that I had. So I eventually stole a prescription pad from one doctor's office; I had his DEA number so I just wrote my own prescriptions for what I wanted. Eventually, I stole other pads from other doctors and hospitals. At one time, I had 30-40 pads from different doctors.

I knew one doctor and one dentist who would give you a prescription, as a kickback, when you made an appointment with them. This, however, was the exception rather than the rule.

I think I had hit about every pharmacy in the metropolitan area. I was worried about getting caught. But of all the prescriptions I got filled, I would say I got turned down only about 1% of the time. And, I don't think I was that good at what I was doing, I just think some pharmacists didn't know what to do with a suspicious prescription. Then, a few pharmacies just turned their heads. I was very comfortable going to some drug stores — I don't know if they just wanted the business or didn't want the hassle of reporting me. But I would go in their stores, often high on drugs; they had to have noticed.

My drug of choice was Demerol which is synthetic morphine. On an average day, I was going through 1,500 milligrams of Demerol. The drug came in 50-milligram and 100-milligram tablets. A typical prescription for bad pain might be one 50-milligram tablet every four hours. So, I'd say a high dosage would be 300 milligrams a day. My habit was progressive, getting worse over time.

It was easy to get drugs. I would get one or two prescriptions a day. My preferred method of using was to inject it. I'd buy a box of needles and would shoot up maybe ten to twelve times a day. I was going through dozens of needles. The veins in my arms and legs were so collapsed the only way I could tap into my vascular system was through my jugular vein. I'd sit in front of a mirror and shoot up through my jugular which had a two-inch by quarter-inch scab over it at that point. I would poke through the scab to inject myself. It was hideous, but I could not stop. I was hauled to the hospital by ambulance several times for overdosing.

My day-to-day life was getting drugs. It was a miserable existence. I lied, cheated. I needed drugs more than food, companionship or shelter. I looked like a cadaver. Everyone around me told me how sick I was and how I needed help. Unfortunately, I was the last one to realize it.

Eventually, I was arrested. I think I must have wanted to get caught and was crying out for help, because toward the end I was using my real name and address when I wrote my own prescriptions.

The day I was arrested, I had gone to the same pharmacy twice in one day to get prescriptions filled. The pharmacist had become suspicious. So when he gave me the second prescription, he gave me only half the pills, explaining that he was out of them and that I'd have to come back for the second half. I thought it might be a set-up, but I was also an addict so I went back later for the second half. I even waited for 30 minutes.

The pharmacist had called the police and they came and arrested me. Initially I was terrified of what was going to happen to me, but at the same time I think there was relief that things were coming to an end. On some level I knew I was very sick and needed help. Anyone living the life I was can expect to sit down to a banquet of consequences. I was long overdue.

I'm now in recovery. I was lucky. I only got probation and did not go to prison. I speak to recovery groups around town. I think very few people have an understanding of the scope of prescription drug abuse and addiction. My case was extreme, but a lot of others are abusing on a lesser level; they think it's okay because it's a prescription.

Turning Point: My arrest. I was looking at a possible 5-10 year jail sentence for obtaining a controlled substance by fraud. That snapped me into reality. It wasn't the physical damage I was doing to myself with the drugs that stopped me — in my own warped mind it was worth it.

Advice to Others: One thing I've learned is that someone who's chemically dependent is not going to take anyone's advice until they're ready. You can give someone advice and talk until you're blue in the face, but until they're ready to help themselves, it's useless. Most people already know, deep down, when they're in trouble — they just won't admit it. Some people have to get cornered, like I did, before they're ready to get help.

Addiction is a progressive disease and it will get worse. And, if you are deeply involved with drugs, like I was, you're going to meet with some kind of tragedy. You've got to reach down deep inside yourself to want to get help. My wish for others is that they can do that without going through what I went through.

Other Factors Influencing Prescription Drug Diversion

In an address to the American Medical Association in 1988, Robert McAfee, MD, noted five factors influencing trends toward abuse of prescription drugs, rather than illicit drugs:

1) **Risk of disease, especially AIDS**. As addicts look for ways to minimize their risk of HIV infection, more users are

turning to prescription drugs because the product is pure, and an oral form can be used rather than an intravenous one. A prime example is the use of Dilaudid instead of injected heroin.

2) **Urine testing by employers.** Often if a job candidate can demonstrate he's taking a prescription drug — and even show the prescription bottle — he's often exempt from negative consequences if a urine test is positive. Sometimes, having a prescription bottle handy will preclude having a urine test altogether.

3) **Drug abusers are more sophisticated.** They learn how to produce certain psychological effects with combinations of pharmaceuticals — drugs which are more predictable in terms of purity, onset and duration of effect.

4) **Lack of stringent drug laws.** In some areas, defrauding physicians or pharmacists is only a misdemeanor, in contrast to the felony offense for dealing with illicit drugs.

5) **Financial gain.** The costs of prescription drugs are often covered through Medicaid or other health insurance. While the addict on the street must produce hard cash to buy an illicit drug such as heroin, a prescription drug abuser may well have his drug of choice paid for through health insurance.

Black Market Drug Sales

Next to nuclear materials, prescription drugs are perhaps the most highly controlled commodity in the world. Still, the DEA estimates that illegal diversion of legally controlled substances constitutes a multi-billion dollar annual market. Unlike the scammers who obtain drugs to self-medicate, those involved in the black market or street sale of pharmaceuticals are out for big money (See Table 10).

For example, a Dilaudid tablet, prescribed for pain, but often referred to as "drug store heroin," by dealers, is one of the most sought-after drugs on the street. It can sell for $60 or more per tablet. A cancer patient might commonly receive a prescription of 200-300 tablets, with a street value of $12,000 to $18,000.

Table 10. Comparative Prices of Popular Controlled Drugs

In order of street user preference:

Name	Pharmacy price per pill	Street Price per pill	% Profit
Dilaudid	$ 2.00	$50-$100.00	2,500%-5,000%
Valium	1.04	6.00	477
Ativan	1.03	5.00	385
Darvocet	.73	2.00	174
Xanax	.79	2.00	153
Sinequan	.51	.75	47
Empirin w/ Codeine	.70	4.00	471
Darvon-N	.70	2.00	186
Librium	.97	2.00	106
Tuinal	.43	8.00	1,760
Seconal	.33	6.00	1,718
Florinal w/Codeine	.90	4.00	344
Biphetamine	2.67	7.00	162
Dexedrine	.13	5.00	3,746
Nembutal	.67	7.00	945
Dalmane	.61	2.00	228
Percocet	.85	5.00	488
Tylenol w/Codeine	.38	3.00	689
Percodan	1.09	7.00	542

Source: From "Medicaid Drug Fraud, Federal Leadership Needed to Reduce Program Vulnerabilities" 1993, U.S. General Accounting Office Report to Congressional Requesters,
GAO/HRD-93-118, p. 36. Washington, D.C., U.S. Government Printing Office, 1993.

In Missouri, narcotics agents traced a professional con artist's tracks after his arrest. Over a year's time, the scammer hit 25 midwest physicians, amassed nearly five thousand doses of Dilaudid and made a net profit of $915,000. Endless sophisticated scams fuel this multi-million dollar industry.

In the "car phone scam," the con artist calls a pharmacy, identifies himself as a doctor calling from his car phone and orders a patient prescription. He tells the pharmacist he'll soon be out of range with his car phone. The caller also tells the pharmacist that he's just received the call on his mobile phone from the patient. Therefore, the con man explains, no one at his office can verify the patient request. This tactic distracts the pharmacist from trying to verify the call immediately.

With the "phoney police officer scam," the offender phones a pharmacy and states that he's a narcotics detective and that a con artist under surveillance is about to approach the pharmacy with a bogus prescription. The "officer" instructs the pharmacist to fill the prescription, explaining that police will then make an arrest. Once the scammer leaves the store, no police ever arrive.

A scam used successfully several times in the Denver area is the "new doctor in town." The defrauder has his own prescription pads printed; the office phone number listed on the pad is actually a public phone booth number. An accomplice takes the prescription in while a partner waits at the phone booth. When the pharmacist calls to verify the prescription, the con artist answers the phone, saying he's the doctor and he approves the transaction.

9 Medicaid Prescription Fraud

You may not know anyone involved in the black marketing of pharmaceuticals, but you, as a taxpayer, are affected by it. Medicaid prescription fraud is conservatively estimated to cost several billion dollars annually, based on statistics generated by individual states.

The opportunities for abuse and fraud of the Medicaid system are many and the profits potentially high, according to the General Accounting Office (GAO). The greater portion of Medicaid fraud occurs at the provider — doctor or pharmacy — levels, although a recipient (patient) is necessarily involved in schemes either knowingly or unknowingly.

The incentives for abuse are derived from two classes of drugs. First, are those many prescription drugs that have effects similar to illicit street drugs (Valium or Ritalin, for example) but may be cheaper or safer to use by the street-level drug abuser. The second class includes other therapeutic drugs that have high dollar values and are diverted for resale back to pharmacies at less than wholesale prices. The sample of convictions reviewed by the GAO in four states involved total billings of $12 million over three years, of which only $280,000 was recovered.

GAO officials point out that fraudulent schemes, large or small, capitalize on weaknesses within the regulatory functions of the Medicaid system. Medicaid's structure and organization, fee-for-service and limited copayments, invite overuse by honest providers and recipients, to say nothing of those with less honest objectives.

Why has this occurred? Leslie G. Arnonvitz, Associate Director, Health Financing Issues of the Health and Human Services Division of the GAO, reports two major reasons: "First, the resources devoted to enforcement activities are very limited in all the jurisdictions. And secondly, the priority in the past to prosecute health fraud has not been very high because of the focus on other types of crime."

Examples of Provider Fraud

Organized drug diversion schemes against Medicaid take several forms. Some of the most common are:

- Pharmacists adding medications to patient prescriptions and keeping the excess for their own use or for resale
- Clinics providing inappropriate prescriptions that are then used by recipients to obtain drugs for resale on the street
- Pharmacies allowing recipients to trade prescriptions for other merchandise sold by the pharmacy
- Pill Mills. In these schemes, physicians provide a medically unnecessary prescription. Then, the recipient sells the prescription to pharmacist or street dealer for cash, merchandise or other abuseable drugs. Then, the pharmacist diverts the prescription for resale and bills Medicaid for the prescription.

In a 1993 GAO study, half of the 42 Medicaid Fraud Control Units contacted reported ongoing investigations of "pill mill" operations. The pill mill cases operated in locations as diverse as New York City and Buckhannon, West Virginia. Remaining states reporting these schemes to the GAO included: California, Texas, Florida, Illinois, Michigan, New Jersey, Massachusetts, Indiana, Washington, Maryland, Minnesota, Louisiana, Kentucky, Oklahoma, Oregon, New Mexico, Rhode Island, Delaware and the District of Columbia.

Forty-two states have Medicaid Fraud Control Units (MFCUs) that investigate fraud within the state's Medicaid agencies. States without MFCU's use local and federal law enforcement to investigate and prosecute Medicaid fraud.

Other Examples of Provider Fraud

- One physician writes 2,000 Medicaid prescriptions in a month.
- A pharmacist bills 30 prescriptions for one recipient in one day.
- In a four-day period, one recipient is given the same lab test five times and has six prescriptions for Zantac filled. (Zantac, an ulcer medication, is very valuable for resale to pharmacies).
- In New York, "patient brokers" recruit homeless and addicted Medicaid recipients, and send them to conspiring clinics that bill for unnecessary tests and give unnecessary prescriptions. These drugs are then resold at less than wholesale prices for resale to pharmacies and are again available for a fraudulent billing to Medicaid.
- Eight Texas physicians, with billings of $11 million dollars in one year, are convicted of drug diversion.

Examples of Recipient Fraud

In California, a senior Medicaid investigator described one suspect who admitted to using his Medi-Cal to pay for his prescriptions and then sell them on the street. His Medi-Cal billing for one year was $28,000.

The same investigator cited other examples. "Another suspect was arrested for doctor shopping. In a five-month period, the subject had 89 prescriptions for Tylenol with Codeine III — prescriptions written by 42 different physicians and filled at 25 pharmacies. The bill was in excess of $8,000."

A third suspect had prescriptions written by 18 doctors, and filled at 22 pharmacies. Upon his arrest, he reported that he was tired of buying Methamphetamine from the street, so he studied medical journals and found he could get a similar high from Ritalin. His Medi-Cal bill was $13,000.

"All these individuals were dealing in prescription controlled substances," the investigator said. "All were on Medi-Cal and were using Medi-Cal to pay for drugs and/or doctors' visits. Their drugs of choice were Codeine, Vicodin, Percodan, Valium and Doriden." Because Medicaid fraud units are understaffed, the investigator also cited a need for keener awareness of the problem by the justice system. "I've done a lot of training for local law enforcement. It's an area of drugs they're just not real familiar with. They don't pay a lot of attention to it. I've had police officers call me and tell me, 'I found a bunch of bottles of this and that. I don't know what it is. What do I do with it?' Most of them ignore it. Perhaps the District Attorneys need the most training. I've heard them say, 'It's only pills'."

Law Enforcement Limitations

Medicaid drug diversions are highly resistant to detection and once detected, to investigation, prosecution, and conviction as well.

For the Medicaid fraud units, the shortages in both technology and personnel take their toll. The system relies on tips and referrals rather than data analysis and intelligence to reveal abuses. Furthermore, the pursuit of fraud cases is hugely labor intensive, the time frames are long and the chances of success are slim. A case in point — in Florida, the GAO learned that because of manpower shortages, Medicaid fraud investigators might investigate only 10% of the complaints of possible fraud on file with the Medicaid providers.

In four other states, 39 cases reviewed showed neither timely nor satisfactory results. Almost half the cases took over two years to resolve; some cases, involving license revocation, lingered for seven years; penalties were mild — few went to jail, and more than half those convicted experienced no licensure action or probation. "It all has to do with how tough it is to prove these cases," explains Aronovitz. "Even once you do prove something, you often only get the low man on the totem pole rather than the corporate entity. The pay off is not there in terms of the amount of time you have to spend investigating fraud."

Solutions to Medicaid Fraud

Given the scope of the problem of prescription drug fraud, states and the federal government have been searching for strategies to stem the hemorrhaging of money from the Medicaid system. These efforts have three broad themes: 1) prevention and detection, 2) administrative sanctions, and 3) recovery and restitution of the money defrauded.

Strategies to Prevent Recipient Fraud

- More stringent identification, including photo ID's with fingerprints included.
- On-line eligibility verification at the time a Medicaid prescription is filled at the pharmacy.
- Establish utilization limits, restricting the number of prescriptions that could be filled in a given period of time, usually per month.
- On line utilization review. An ID card would be like a "credit card" and the recipient's prescription usage would be analyzed immediately at the point of sale. Any unusual or abuse-like trends would immediately prevent the filling of that prescription.
- Post and clear systems. "Post and clear" refers to an on-line system which tracks a prescription from the time it's written to the time it is filled at the pharmacy. Diversion along the way is more difficult.

State efforts at pursuit and punishment of drug diversion provider networks are also becoming more aggressive with efforts to halt the profitability of fraudulent schemes and to punish or jeopardize the professional standing of the providers involved.

As Aronovitz suggests, "It's in everyone's best interest that Medicaid fraud be stopped. When a program is vulnerable to fraud, it's not the program that pays back money lost…it's the taxpayers. It's something everyone needs to be concerned about. We're all being hurt by it, we just don't realize it."

PART THREE

Toward Solutions

10 Education... First Line of Defense

"Prescription drug abuse is the least understood, least discussed and possibly the most disgraceful part of the nation's drug problem. We know how to fix it but we lack the will and the resources," explains Bonnie Wilford, Director, Pharmaceutical Policy Research Center George Washington University. "If we can't solve this problem, which we can monitor, how can we ever solve the illegal drug problem?" Indeed, public education will be a driving force in the development of resources for curtailing pharmaceutical diversion.

In the commentaries that follow, substance abuse experts, physicians and educators offer opinions on improving education for both health care professionals and consumers.

David E. Smith, MD, President
American Society Addiction Medicine
San Francisco, California

We need much greater public awareness about prescription drug abuse. The country's addiction problems with all substances — alcohol, tobacco, illegal drugs and legal drugs represent one of our most serious health hazards. The consequences of untreated substance abuse include traffic accidents and other trauma, poor health, AIDS, family disintegration, dropping out of school, joblessness, underemployment, worker absenteeism and reduced worker productivity.

The financial toll for substance abuse is staggering. The costs of tobacco, alcohol and other drug abuse in the United States exceeds $238 billion a year.

There's a human toll, too. Over a half million people die every year because of substance abuse. About 50% of all preventable deaths are related to some aspect of substance abuse. One out of every five hospital beds is occupied by somebody with substance abuse as a contributing factor.

When it comes to long-term abuse of prescription drugs, there's no question that there is a cumulative effect, and it can reduce life expectancy by about fifteen years. In addition, we're also seeing a growing trend toward the abuse of multiple drugs — both illegal and legal. We see a lot of narcotics being mixed with alcohol. As a nation, we take prescription drug abuse too lightly as a health issue. If it's not cocaine or some other street drug, we don't think of it as a problem.

Still, treating substance abuse not only saves lives, but saves dollars. A study by the National Institute on Drug Abuse found that each dollar spent on addiction treatment saved $4 to $7 in reduced medical and social costs, and returned $3 in increased worker productivity. The study concluded that each $1 invested in treatment returns $7 to $10 to society.

Thomas D. Wyatt, Executive Director
National Association of State Controlled
Substances Authorities
Columbia, South Carolina

It's hard to nail down a solution to such a complex problem. Altogether, prescription drug abuse, misuse and addiction is a pervasive problem. The laws are adequate, but operationally they're hard to enforce on many levels. For example, it's illegal to trade prescriptions with your neighbor, but few people are going to get arrested for that.

Public education is critical, but it's a complex issue and you can't explain it in five minutes. Education for professionals is important. For example, I'm a pharmacist and an attorney. I do about 35 hours of mandatory continuing education training a year to keep my licenses. But, many states have no required continuing education for physicians. Only certain doctors who are members of certain colleges or who are specialists are required to update their training.

I think the main safeguard against becoming an unwitting addict is having a knowledgeable doctor. One of the big problems is that we don't have enough addiction training for doctors in medical schools.

However, if you're going to educate a physician in five years of medical school, you can't touch on everything. Doctors can get some education on a voluntary basis after med school, but most of them are too busy. Most doctors care a great deal, they're just too busy.

Clearly, there are many good doctors and many good drugs. There is a perfectly good use for many of these drugs which have addiction potential. They need to be properly used.

Monitoring systems, such as electronic monitoring, can help curb abuse, but some states have a paranoia about privacy, saying that monitoring violates a patient's right to privacy. But you can't have your cake and eat it, too. Perhaps we can eventually have a monitoring system that protects privacy, yet is open enough to tell us if John Doe is buying drugs under another name, for example.

I also think the regulatory people, federal and state, get a lot of bashing they don't deserve. They're often seen by marketing people as obstructing the free marketing of drugs.

For example, regulators in New York got a lot of flack when they cracked down on benzodiazepines. (They required that the prescriptions be issued in triplicate, with a copy going to the state for monitoring purposes.) There was a lot of weeping and wailing from manufacturers and the American Medical Association, complaining that bad drugs would be used in their place. But that just hasn't happened, nor has there been any breech of confidentiality with a patient's name.

Jeff Baldwin, PharmD
Associate Professor of Pharmacy
University of Nebraska College of Pharmacy
Omaha, Nebraska

Many medical professionals, including pharmacists, don't know what to do about addictions. Most medical schools and pharmacy schools do a lousy job teaching about addiction.

I chair the Substance Abuse Special Interest Group in the American Association of Colleges of Pharmacy, and can speak directly to the issue of educating of pharmacists. Our special interest group is made up of pharmacy college faculty who, among other things, are pushing for required courses on substance abuse. We've done surveys of pharmacy students and colleges and found that very few have information about addiction or substance abuse in their course of study. Part of that is because the faculty themselves have not been taught about it.

We do a good job of teaching students about the pharmacology of drugs, which is how drugs work in the body. And we teach about the toxicology of drugs, that is, what happens when you overdose. But we don't teach students the psychosocial aspects which is basically what the drug does to the person — how it interacts with perception, personality and behavior.

Recently, for the first time at our college, we have a required course on substance abuse for first year students. It deals with the more human aspects of addiction, rather than the scientific. As part of the course, I require each student to attend a 12-step meeting so they can see what support groups are about.

Pharmacy needs to move toward "pharmaceutical care," in which the pharmacist has a greater role in the patient's therapy, seeing the scripts are refilled appropriately and not over-used.

David Mee-Lee, MD (ASAM)
Castle Medical Center
Honolulu, Hawaii

In general, I think doctors have not been given the training to deal with addiction; however, that is changing slowly — medical schools are starting to offer coursework. But I think physicians' attitudes are simply a reflection of society's view that addiction is a moral problem or shows lack of willpower. Addicts are often seen as people who are out of control rather than as having an illness. If you break your leg and are off work for three weeks, people see that differently than if you've spent three weeks in a drug rehab program.

On top of that mindset, because doctors see the same addicts over and over in emergency rooms, physicians might start feeling that some of these people are hopeless, that they're not trying to get better. Then, if a doctor never goes to an AA meeting to see people in recovery, he or she can slip into a negative attitude about addiction. Doctors need to have a better understanding of addiction, do better monitoring of patients and better screening for addiction risk factors. They also need to know how to direct patients into recovery.

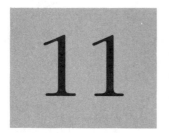

11 Drug Manufacturers' Role in Consumer Education

Drug manufacturers — the ones producing high-powered narcotics — do they have a role in educating consumers about a drug's potential for abuse? Or is that a role belonging only to the prescriber? Are pharmaceutical companies responsible for efforts to curb diversion?

Can the companies be held responsible for drug abuse beyond the point of sale, when the drug is in the hands of consumers? Does a drug manufacturer's for-profit motive imply disinterest in drug products being abused?

In the following commentaries, representatives from the drug industry respond to charges leveled by some health care and regulatory professionals who say the industry shows a lack of concern about drug abuse and diversion.

Thomas D. Wyatt, Executive Director
National Association State Controlled
Substances Authorities

The pharmaceutical companies have a role in consumer education. They don't like me very much because I'm pretty vocal in my opinion that they need to reduce their marketing effort and focus more on education. But the focus is the bottom line. They all give lip service to public education, but there's a big difference in the amount of dollars they spend on marketing drugs and the amount they spend on education.

Scott Nelson, Manager Public Affairs
DuPont-Merck Pharmaceutical Company
Wilimington, Delaware

I could build a case that our marketing is about education. Our reps go into doctors' offices and do a combination of sales work and education. The people in this business — and it is a business — have an interest in business on the one hand and also genuinely believe that our products can be helpful when used appropriately. These products save lives, eliminate suffering.

I will also say that I do not believe our sales reps mislead physicians. Any drug rep knows he or she can mislead a customer once and make a sale, but it kills sales in the long run. Misuse of drugs is in no one's best interest. Not the patient's. Not the doctor's. Not our drug company's. If a patient has a bad experience with our product, it's likely a doctor will not prescribe it again. If a drug develops a reputation as having high potential for abuse, doctors really become reluctant to prescribe it.

On the issue of diversion, we take many measures, prescribed by state and federal law, through our manufacturing and distribution process, to prevent diversion. Our internal safeguards are many. People who work in our manufacturing plants are all drug-tested before they're employed and their backgrounds are checked for any drug-related offenses. If employees work with controlled substances, they can have no pockets in their uniforms. Any Schedule II or III drugs are kept in a vault in our distribution center; all products are logged in and out. Every single tablet must be accounted for. Then, drugs can be shipped only with bonded carriers. The controls at our level are much more stringent than at the retail pharmacy level.

When it comes to the individual who is obtaining pharmaceuticals illegally, we cooperate with authorities. We see this crime as out of our scope of authority. We have, however, worked very hard to promote the appropriate use of our medications when we talk with health care professionals. We have 400 reps out there, talking to doctors. These drugs are the tools of their trade; my experience is that doctors become educated on the drugs they prescribe. We can get in to see physicians, although the doctors probably have less time to spend with us now than they did ten years ago.

Historically, we have not communicated directly with consumers. The FDA has discouraged our speaking directly to patients, and so have physicians. The doctors prefer to maintain the stronger bond between themselves and the patient. We haven't done direct-to-consumer promotions. Our marketing is directed at health care professionals. And frankly, it's probably not appropriate for us to advertise or promote controlled substances. We would be perceived as irresponsible.

However, just in the last couple of years we have started communicating directly with consumers; an example is our ad for Proscar, a drug for men with enlarged prostate glands. But that's a far different drug than a controlled substance. I think there's a trend toward more consumer education. We are not planning, at any level, to actively promote our controlled substances, Percodan and Percocet, at this point. They're rather late in their product life cycle.

From the corporate point of view, I think the most frustrating thing is that people tend to lump appropriate use and misuse together.

We would like patients to benefit from the appropriate use of our medication, but when others use pharmaceuticals for nonmedical reasons it gives the drugs a bad name. And, it often makes people who are legitimately using these feel like their use is inappropriate, too.

Ronald Gershman, MD (ASAM)
Los Angeles, California

The pharmaceutical companies have a big role in the abuse/misuse problem. Without a question, they mislead doctors as to the hazards of addiction and abuse of their medications. It's a strong statement, but it exists, unequivocally.

Doctors cannot get the level of education they need about a drug from a sales rep from a for-profit corporation.

Tom
Pharmaceutical sales rep, 17 years

Some sales reps do mislead physicians. They might not explain to doctors the drug's side effects. They mislead them on prices. Some sales people will make up answers to questions. There's no justification for this, but it happens. Eventually the dishonest rep gets caught, then physicians will have nothing to do with him or her. Then, it hurts the whole industry.

I've stayed in business as long as I have by just being honest. If I don't know the answer to a question, I tell them I don't know. I don't bash other companies' products, I just tell my customers the benefits of mine.

In some markets it's easy to talk to doctors, to educate them. In some markets it's difficult. In one of the cities I serve it's almost impossible to see physicians. They just refuse to see us drug reps. The doctors in that particular town also have a more blasé attitude about scheduled drugs. These doctors' knowledge of some of our products suffers.

The pharmaceutical industry does push sales, but in addition to trying to make sales, you're trying to educate your customers. If health professionals are not educated about the drug, they'll eventually quit using it. So it's important that they know about it. Pharmaceutical companies have a role in consumer education. We've started trying to help educate physicians about addiction as well as scammers. We put out a packet of information for doctors, including a log sheet for use in keeping track of samples. We also distribute patient brochures, but I think most of them get tossed in the garbage.

Some companies are very conscientious about the education of doctors and patients. Other companies focus on profit. Most of us reps know which is which. Most doctors don't.

I think drug manufacturers should do away with free samples to physicians, but I don't think it will happen. If doctors have samples, they'll usually write prescriptions for the drug. But scheduled samples are a mess. They're easily stolen in many offices. We manufacture one of the most highly-diverted prescription drugs. I won't have samples sent to a doctor's office unless I know they keep them under lock and track them with a written log.

Doctors are required by law to report only drug thefts over $500. That leaves a lot of room for crimes of theft to go unreported.

Jeff Newton, Director Media Relations
Eli Lilly & Company
Indianapolis, Indiana

As a company, we're dedicated to making life-saving medications. We, along with other manufacturers, have been very successful at it. These drugs only complete their mission of saving lives and helping people if they're used properly and prescribed properly. Patient compliance is key to the drug's success.

We are a private business and we do have a revenue stream. But consider that it costs around $350 million to develop a new drug; it's not government money we're investing, it's company dollars. So yes, we're in business to make money.

Still, education about how to use Lilly products (among them Darvon and Darvocet) is a high corporate priority. Our sales reps are highly trained to fully understand our products and how they are used; reps can promote a certain drug for only the specific indications approved by the FDA.

We do no direct-to-consumer advertising for any of our products. However, in addition to working with doctors, we work closely with the pharmacy community and make sure they have knowledge about our drugs.

We also have at our headquarters phone banks, people working in customer service, who take phone calls from health professionals as well as consumers. These people working in customer services are also highly trained.

Unfortunately, prescription drug abuse can result in a lack of public awareness that manufacturers invent these drugs to provide a tremendous human benefit. We're about saving lives, not just making pills. But so many times, we see a story about a problem with a drug, the maker is named and it casts a shadow.

Jeff Trewitt, Vice President for Communications
Pharmaceutical Research
and Manufacturers of America (PhRMA)
Washington, D.C.

PhRMA is the national trade association for over 100 research-based pharmaceutical companies in the United States. The organization serves as the pharmaceutical industry's voice on policy issues concerning health care reform, regulation by the FDA, research from the National Institutes of Health and health care bills.

Traditionally, pharmaceutical companies have contributed to consumer education by making doctors aware of what they need to know about the safe use of drugs. The physician, in turn, is supposed to pass on any warnings and advice to patients. The package inserts that accompany medications also provide information for physicians and patients. However, the concept of reaching patients only through physicians is changing somewhat and is being re-evaluated by companies today. More and more companies are trying to provide consumer information themselves through brochures, publications and videos. Companies are holding internal seminars, asking themselves if they should be doing more consumer education. The answer from many companies is "yes." The companies want sales, but they also want good reputations and trust among doctors and patients. On the other hand, many companies would say that they've already covered their responsibilities by providing detailed information in the patient-package insert.

Ed Polich, Director External Affairs
Whitby Pharmaceuticals, Inc./UCB Pharma
Richmond, Virginia

As a company, we are most concerned about pharmaceutical diversion. We have a product, Lortab, a hydrocodone derivative, a Schedule III narcotic. There are tremendously legitimate uses for this drug, and we take enormously stringent internal control measures with these drugs. We don't want to see these drugs going into the wrong hands, but we know it happens.

Another thing that happens when the public hears about legitimate drugs being abused — they become fearful of using a drug that may truly help them. Doctors may also have a knee-jerk response and be afraid to prescribe certain drugs.

So we've asked ourselves what social responsibilities do we have in fighting diversion? What can we do to educate the pharmacists, the prescribers? How we can help medical staffs spot the scammers?

We've taken several measures. We send out newsletters, describing ways to curb vulnerability to scams. We've developed video tapes on addiction recovery issues. We've polled pharmacists about what they thought could be done to stem diversion. They told us they needed more education about identifying scammers and forged prescriptions. We put together a "reduce abuse package" or tip sheet for pharmacists to use in spotting scammers. We've also developed what we call a drug-dispensing register we provide to physicians. We found a lot of practitioners have little education on proper record-keeping and storage of narcotics. This system helps health professionals establish an inventory control as well as internal office security. It certainly thwarts any internal theft, and it also keeps close track of which drugs patients are receiving. Any irregularities can be noticed.

Thousands of doctors we serve have incorporated this system. Many of them have told us they prefer to be in control of tracking their patients' prescriptions rather than turning it over to a bureaucratic agency.

There's nothing wrong with free enterprise, but we have tried to take responsible actions along with our marketing efforts. Not all companies share the same values when it comes to issues of revenue and education.

David
Pharmaceutical sales rep, eight years

Drug companies have a responsibility to provide education, especially to the medical community. And they do that — manufacturers report on their clinical trials — telling what dosages are safe according to FDA guidelines, what the side effects are. Although over the years, some drug companies may have caused a few of their own problems by not being as thorough with reporting as they could have been.

We reps are responsible for informing doctors about a product, and sometimes getting in to see doctors can be difficult. It's a time problem. There are a lot of drugs and a lot of drug company reps. Physicians don't always have time to see all these reps; the doctors often have to rely on brochures we leave for them.

Still, when it comes to prescription drug abuse, I think a lot of entities have to take some responsibility. Manufacturers. Doctors. Patients. It would also help to have better communication between patients and their physicians.

Our company is very cautious about the handling of controlled substances from the point of manufacture to the wholesale warehouse. But once the drugs reach the wholesaler and then are distributed to the retail outlets, there's really no way we can be held accountable for what prescription a physician writes or what the patient does with those pills after receiving them.

Bob Lutz, Director, Business Planning and Development
Knoll Pharmaceutical Co.
Mt. Olive, New Jersey

Among the products we manufacture are two narcotic analgesics (Dilaudid and Vicodin), and we are very active in attempting to minimize the amount of illegal diversion of these products. Legally, we do all that's required to control our products; however, we also assume a moral responsibility to help do what we can to see that these drugs end up where they're supposed to, ultimately in the hands of patients who need them. The mandate that I have from the president of our company is to work with state agencies and professional associations in efforts to minimize diversion.

When we learned about some of the scams being used on doctors and pharmacists to obtain drugs, such as Knoll's, we put together a program to help inform doctors and pharmacists. We felt providing more education to health professionals was the way we could have the most impact, and we think our efforts have made a difference.

When it comes to drug companies making revenue, I don't think there's anything wrong with the free enterprise system. And when our drugs are abused, it might mean a rise in sales for a couple of years, but then that drug is going to drop out of use. Doctors will be afraid to prescribe it if it gets a bad reputation. The example that comes to mind is Methaqualone or Quaalude which is now an illegal drug. It had some value or the FDA wouldn't have approved it, but the drug was so oversold and over-abused, it was taken off the market. A company owes it to itself, its shareholders and to the public to do what it can to fight diversion.

Do drug manufacturers spend a lot of money on marketing? Yes, we do. But a lot of that marketing is educational. It's tough to divorce the two concepts. We make sure our reps tell doctors how to properly use the drugs; otherwise, we end up with problems and lose business. If a rep is over-zealous and misleads prescribers, we're going to hear about it, and so will the FDA.

When we look at prescription drug abuse or diversion as a whole, a lot of elements have part of the responsibility. Some drug companies may have waited too long to recognize this problem. The federal government is not always on top of the situation. We weren't made aware by government investigators that our products were being diverted — and our competitors have told me the same thing — until some state authorities informed us. Federal agencies can become really backlogged with work. Some federal and state officials will say, "The drug you make is being abused, let's put it in another schedule so it will be harder to get." But this is not looking at the core problem. If the scammers can't get a drug because control has been tightened, they're just going to go for another drug.

We also realize that some prescribers aren't skilled at recognizing scams. Pharmacists, too, often need more training in spotting scams. So, everyone is well-intentioned, but there are problems up and down the system. I don't think any one is to blame, yet everyone is to blame, might be one way to say it.

12 Law Enforcement's Dilemma

In this chapter, you'll hear from state and federal law enforcement officers from various corners of the nation; they speak out about the problem of prescription drugs in their regions and, given their resources, what they can and cannot do about it.

Billy S. Allsbrook, Assistant Director
Bureau of Criminal Investigation
Virginia State Police
Richmond, Virginia

Historically, law enforcement's role in fighting prescription drug diversion has been one of reaction, rather than being proactive. A lot of states react on a case by case basis. And, there are some agencies within our state that don't think that this is a significant problem. But it's like opening Pandora's box — once you get the lid off you see how much of a problem it is.

There are other factors for this lack of focus on the problem. Mainly, the resources have gone to fighting illegal drugs while prescription drug diversion gets put on the back burner.

However, we've had the resources to make our Diversion Investigative Unit proactive. We have a staff of 12 people, and take a two-pronged approach in dealing with the problem. First, we investigate violations of the law. That covers illegal activities ranging from people forging prescriptions to patients doctor shopping. Secondly, we focus on continuing education for health professionals. Between 1992 and 1994, our Diversion Investigative Unit conducted 105 educational programs, reaching 4,639 participants — hospital employees, administrators, doctors, nurses and pharmacists. We let these professionals know about the ways in which scammers are trying to dupe them.

The health professionals have been very receptive to our message. The Virginia Hospital Association and the Virginia Insurance Reciprocal have set up seminars. We're also doing classes at the medical college.

Arrests in Virginia for diversion have doubled in the last five years. That's in part because more health professionals are recognizing diversion and reporting it.

It's a growing problem. States need to take a look at it because it's out there.

Michael Moy, Chief
Drug Operations Section
Drug Enforcement Administration (DEA)
Washington, D.C.

Pharmaceutical diversion has been a problem for a number of years. We've been taking increased action against it over the past five to 10 years. However, until we have changes in federal law, we can't do a lot more than we're doing.

We have limited resources, around 420 investigators, so in the DEA we basically target only the major organizations. We take action against someone for diversion 700 to 800 times a year. And, in 80% to 90% of our cases, we coordinate with a number of other agencies at the federal level — the FBI, they have the same authority as DEA.

We may also work with states, many of which now have dedicated programs toward drug diversion. Many states are active. At the local level, some police departments have dedicated units that recognize that pharmaceutical drug diversion is a major problem. In many of the cases we investigate, we use undercover agents or we'll have an informant we recruited.

One of our recent cases involved a script fraud ring. These people were duplicating prescription pads. They were then forging prescriptions and passing them at different pharmacies. They were amassing a lot of drugs. These people were more of the criminal element. Once search warrants were issued, we found a lot of weapons, so it could have become a violent situation.

Are there black market professional rings? Yes. We've got situations where people will go out and recruit "patients," with previous medical problems to go to physicians. Through the physicians, the recruits get prescriptions for certain narcotics. Then, the organizers have the patients fill the prescriptions at pharmacies and sell the drugs on the streets. The organizers then split some of the profits with the so-called patients. They become pretty sophisticated.

In one case, we investigated a physician who was dispensing in excess of a million dosage units of narcotics and benzodiazepines. In this scheme, "patients" would pay the doctor or his staff $50 in cash per visit; often the patients didn't even see the doctor. But the patients would be given multiple prescriptions each day. The patients would not be given refills and they would have to return to his office and pay an additional $50. Some "patients" were reselling the drugs while others used the drugs themselves.

In this case, we coordinated efforts with a local police department, the IRS and the state's health department. There are a number of reasons for including so many agencies. For instance, the doctor in this case had a number of licenses. He had a DEA registration. In some states, doctors are issued two registrations in the state — one to practice medicine and one to handle controlled substances. So in the case of a doctor, if we go in with a variety of agencies that have jurisdiction and authority, then we're able to simultaneously take the doctor's DEA registration and any state registrations. We put them out of business.

Most of these investigations have to take place over a period of time. We're often dealing with health professionals, and often there's a reluctance by people in the community to judge the health professionals guilty of any criminal offenses. In fact, we've had cases where we took action, along with the state, against a doctor's DEA registration, but then the doctor was only put on probation. Then, in a short period of time, the doctor was back in operation. We've received some criticism for having a "chilling effect" on doctors legitimately prescribing controlled substances. But that's rubbish. We do not tell doctors how to practice medicine or try to limit their use of appropriate narcotics. Cracking down on the illegitimate use of legal drugs is our only interest.

Looking at where most of the diversion occurs, we don't find that it clusters in any given part of the United States. It's all over. Of course, major cities like LA, New York, Detroit and Miami have higher rates, but we also investigate rural America as well. The diversion knows no geographical boundaries. Our automated system, known as ARCOS — Automation of Reports and Consolidated Orders System — shows distribution of controlled substances, so we know where medications are being shipped. We can track controlled substances from the point of manufacture to the point of sale. And we have suspect areas throughout the country.

The limitation of our system is, however, that it does not provide data from the prescriber or patient level. Individual prescribers or doctor-shoppers involved in diversion cannot be traced through ARCOS.

Why has there been an increase in this diversion? One reason is that hard-core addicts can get no better "quality control" than with pharmaceuticals. They know it's factory-made and pure. Some prefer it over street drugs.

For the unwitting, the ones who get addicted unknowingly and then don't want to give up the drug, the problem is more hidden because the drugs came from legitimate doctors. To combat the problem we need greater public awareness. People need to know that prescription drug abuse can be as serious as using illegal drugs. We all have a role in understanding the problem — education for schools and the public, law enforcement, health professionals. It's a multifaceted problem.

Sgt. Ritch Wagner
Investigative Services, Nebraska State Patrol
Omaha, Nebraska

We've been able to give drug diversion some priority, but it's more on a case by case basis. It is in our five-year plan for resources, manpower and training. However, we still have other responsibilities, too. For example, if we're in the middle of a homicide investigation, that case gets the priority. But I'd say diversion investigation is about half my case load.

There's no doubt the problem is out there. Any law enforcement agency that looks into it will find they have a diversion problem.

Once a law enforcement agency recognizes the problem exists, it needs to establish rapport with health care professionals — clinics, doctors, hospitals — to let them know help from law enforcement is available. As a result, health professionals will report more fraud.

In the past, health care professionals didn't always know they could get help from law enforcement. When you talk to health professionals, they will tell you this diversion has always been a problem. But they just saw coping with it as the normal course of doing business — they've always had certain people trying to dupe them and always will. But once the health professionals start reporting it, we can do something about it. If they don't report, we won't know about it.

I'd say over 80% of the diversion we investigate is related to those seeking drugs for self-medication. Primarily these people have had some kind of medical problem that got them into an addictive pattern with prescription drugs. So then they go beyond legitimate usage and it gets out of hand.

All too often, people don't realize how serious this drug use can be. They don't realize part of the reason some of these drugs are controlled by the federal government is because they are potentially addictive.

In one case, we were twice called to a local hospital, where drugs were disappearing from the pharmacy. With the help of the health department, we identified a pharmacist who had taken over 4,000 dosage units in a year and a half.

I once arrested a certified medical assistant who was working in a doctor's office. She had migraine headaches over the past year and had started stealing sample drugs as well as writing her own prescriptions for Fiorinal with Codeine on the doctor's pads.

I arrested another woman three separate times. She was a nursing assistant in a nursing home. She may have been diverting drugs from the nursing home, but she was also dentist shopping. She did have a dental problem, but she used that as an excuse and went from dentist to dentist to get Tylenol with Codeine.

We arrested her once and she was placed in pre-trial diversion, meaning if she completed her 12-month probation, the charges would be dropped. It really gave her a break. The week after she was placed on pre-trial diversion, we arrested her again for more doctor shopping. This time she was put on two years probation. Eventually, I arrested her a third time for the same thing. The last time I arrested her she looked at me and said, "I've got a problem. I can't do it by myself."

She did go into a rehab center.

We also know there are groups diverting for street resale. Ritalin and Talwin are popular drugs. But in this state it is a limited market and a very closed group, hard to get into. We even know who some of the people involved are, but in order to infiltrate the groups, it takes such a devotion of man hours. It's really too labor intensive to try to break it.

Joanne Schuler, Investigator
Tennessee Bureau of Investigation,
Nashville, Tennessee

We have 18 agents who handle drug cases statewide. I'm the only one who investigates prescription drug diversion. It is a common problem both in the metropolitan and rural areas. Tennessee is primarily a rural state, and I cover cases from Memphis to Mountain City. I've had one case where a woman was going from one doctor to another in rural counties. These kinds of drug problems are no longer confined to the cities.

We have the diversion by individual doctor shoppers as well as that by professionals such as doctors, nurses or pharmacists. Because of lack of resources and investigators, we mostly go after the provider fraud — the health professionals who are diverting. We had to make a decision on what would be most productive, given the resources we have.

Plus, we don't have terribly stringent laws to address the problem of doctor shopping in this state. Unless we can pin down forgeries, as in forged prescriptions, it's hard to pursue.

When we do go after professionals, it can get very complicated because we have to involve the state health boards. Sometimes it's hard to draw the line between what might be intentional overprescribing or incompetence on the physician's part. At the same time, it's very important, from an investigative viewpoint, that I work with the state agencies, the board of pharmacy and the DEA because these cases involving professionals can be difficult to pinpoint. We need a lot of resources to detect wrongdoing.

I think health professionals who are diverting drugs should be taken as seriously as those individuals who are selling street drugs. I worked with Medicaid fraud for a number of years, and the health professionals who were caught diverting rarely got much punishment. We tend to look at these people much differently than those dealing street drugs, and I think in some ways, it's more serious. The professionals have had the training — they know the dangers, but yet they do it.

I think the reason the illicit drug trafficking has gotten more attention is because it usually involves more violence or potential for violence. The public needs to be more concerned about pharmaceutical diversion, but people just aren't aware of the degree to which the average Joe can become hooked on legal drugs and then begin to violate the law to get what he needs.

Bonnie Wilford, Director
Pharmaceutical Policy Research Center
George Washington University
Washington, D.C.

The justice system operates reasonably well in terms of the systems that examine new drugs as they come onto the market and assign schedules to them. But one of the areas for improvement is investigations. We need more investigators with adequate training.

The justice system also has problems with its backlog of cases. In the case of health professionals who have been charged with wrong-doing...they can often continue operating for a number of years before their cases wind their way through the appeal process. So, we can have the best investigators in the world, and there are many fine ones out there, but if the results of an investigation sit in a court docket pending appeal for years, the system has broken down.

Model State Drug Laws

The President's Commission on Model State Drug Laws was formed in 1992 to help states develop laws to fight the drug crisis in America. The 24 commissioners appointed by the Bush Administration included state legislators, treatment service providers, police chiefs, state attorneys general, a housing specialist, district attorneys, a state judge, prevention specialists, attorneys, an urban mayor and other experts. This bipartisan commission was formed as a response to concerns that state governments were addressing the problems of drugs without sufficient planning.

The Commission continued under the Clinton Administration, becoming the National Alliance for Model State Drug Laws. Formed in October 1993, the Alliance's board represents 17 states and the District of the Columbia.

The work of the alliance has been to develop comprehensive model state laws to reduce alcohol and other drug abuse through prevention, education, treatment, enforcement and corrections.

For six months, commission task forces held public hearings to gather information on the efforts of successful individuals, programs and policies. After intensive review and analysis of the testimony, the commission presented its five-volume final report which included 42 model state laws and two policy statements. Issues addressed in their comprehensive report included: economic remedies; community mobilization; crimes code enforcement; alcohol and other drug treatment; and drug-free families, schools and work places.

To ensure the Commission's recommendations were practical, much of the model legislation was based upon legislation and programs implemented in various states throughout the country. In issuing its final report, the Commission offered a blueprint for states to address their alcohol and other drug abuse problems. The model laws were first made available in January 1994 for states to consider. States could tailor any portion of the laws to meet their specific needs. The resulting legislation would then be introduced to state legislatures for passage.

Although the Model State Drug Laws offered a portfolio of legislative initiatives focused on helping states curb the abuse of alcohol and illegal drugs, the problems of prescription drugs did not go unnoticed. "Prescription drug abuse is a problem of epidemic proportion," states Sherry Green, Executive Director of the National Alliance for Model State Drug Laws. Therefore, the Alliance also drafted the Model Prescription Accountability Act, designed to stop diversion of pharmaceuticals, without impeding legitimate prescribing.

At the heart of the Model Prescription Accountability Act was the recommendation for an electronic monitoring system

— electronic data transfer — which would collect information on doctors, pharmacists and patients receiving controlled substances, and compare it with programmed criteria to detect suspicious prescriptions.

The Commission on Model Drug Laws has provided a foundation for states to build upon their efforts to combat drug abuse and its devastating personal and societal effects. But for the Commission's recommendations to bear fruit, the states must be committed to recognizing and solving this problem, Green said. "The use of the Model Drug Laws is in its infancy in the sense that more states need to be doing something with this system. We've provided a framework. All states need to address the issue."

13 Diversion Control Systems

In most states, when you receive a prescription for a drug, the matter is between you, your doctor and your pharmacist. However, in 11 states prescriptions for certain controlled substances are monitored; the intent is to detect excessive amounts of drugs such as narcotics being received by one individual or being prescribed by one health professional.

Most states with monitoring systems use a Multiple Copy Prescription Program (MCPP); three states use Electronic Data Transfer (EDT).

Multiple Copy Prescription Programs

Under Multiple Copy Prescription Programs, practitioners, including physicians, dentists, podiatrists, nurse practitioners and veterinarians, are provided with state-issued triplicate prescription forms. Once a prescription is written, the doctor keeps one copy; the patient takes two copies to the pharmacy which keeps a copy and passes the third copy on to a designated state agency. There, the data is entered into a computer system, so that any irregular practices such as over-prescribing or use of multiple doctors by a patient can be detected and reported.

To date, nine states have some form of triplicate systems in place: New York, California, Idaho, Texas, Illinois, Michigan, Rhode Island, Washington and Hawaii. (Hawaii uses a duplicate system in tandem with a voluntary computerized system.)

Opposition to MCPP monitoring has traditionally come from the medical community and pharmaceutical manufacturers. DEA officials suggest that manufacturers oppose monitoring because of the negative impact on sales. Manufacturers argue that doctors are discouraged from prescribing drugs to patients with legitimate needs for the medication. Many physicians dislike being "watched" by agencies whose personnel are not trained in drug-therapy. Still other critics are concerned that monitoring systems can lead to the inappropriate investigation of legitimate patients; for example, computer tabulations on prescriptions for a patient, suffering from cancer and taking large doses of opioids, could identify the patient as an abuser.

In New York state, the triplicate system has not been without controversy and legal challenges. Legislators first passed laws to establish the triplicate prescription program in 1972; however, due to subsequent legal challenges to the legislation putting Schedule II drugs on triplicate, the program was not fully implemented until 1978.

Then, controversy flared again in 1981, when New York sought to put benzodiazepines under the triplicate system. Implementation was delayed by a succession of court actions to block the new regulation by four drug manufacturers and the New York Medical Society. Consequently, the measure did not go into effect until 1989.

Nonetheless, the program is lauded by the New York Department of Public Health.

John Eadie, Director
Division of Public Health Protection
New York Department of Health
Albany, New York

The history of the triplicate program has been one which has demonstrated a dramatic decrease in the abuse of controlled substances, without adversely impacting legitimate prescriptions for controlled substances.

Amphetamines were historically very heavily abused in New York state; however, once they were placed on the triplicate prescription system, within a few short years the volume of prescribing those drugs was reduced by 94% and the abuse, as measured by drug overdoses in hospital emergency rooms, was reduced by 94%.

Likewise, in the case of the barbiturates, we have seen a similar reduction, 95% in prescriptions, as well as an equivalent reduction in overdoses.

Both these results were achieved quickly after the implementation of the triplicate prescription system. And on the contrary, certain drugs like Percodan and Dilaudid, which are used in the treatment of cancer pain and other significant pain, have basically been stable throughout the entire history of the program, and that is because in New York State those drugs were not subject to abuse when the triplicate system came into effect.

We have been able to keep them out of the abuse ever since, which means that the prescribing of those drugs has been basically unaffected. Physicians are using them now as frequently as they did when the program started.

We placed benzodiazepines on triplicates because they were being heavily abused and misprescribed in terms of overuse, perhaps both intentional and unintentional. The result of the regulation has been a significant reduction in benzodiazepine prescribing without having, as far as we can see, any adverse effect on physicians' practice or upon the prescribing alternative drugs. In the first year of the program, benzodiazepine prescribing decreased 44.2% while in the entire United States, prescribing dropped only 9.8%. Emergency room mentions for benzodiazepines in Buffalo and New York City declined 39%; the national mentions for benzodiazepines remained unchanged.

We also eliminated a lot of abuse of these drugs through the Medicaid system. We tracked a group of 3,400 patients who were in the Medicaid Program and who were receiving about 20,000 benzodiazepines a month, about a quarter million a year. Imagine, that many doses for only 3,400 patients! Within five months of the regulation being in effect, their monthly prescription had dropped by 95%.

Another indicator of our success has been the street prices for diverted benzodiazepines, which have increased anywhere from two to five times. This is clearly an indicator of the restrictions applied.

A third indicator was the study we did in pharmacies across the state. Some of these we picked specifically because we had suspicions of them being involved in aggressive pill mill type activities in which they were joining with medical practices and intentionally diverting these drugs to the street. In these pharmacies in the study, within one month, we saw a 76% decline in the number of prescriptions they were issuing, and that was sustained four months later. We also monitored other pharmacies around the state — we saw decline but nothing of that magnitude.

The Commission of Substance Abuse Services of the state has periodically done a survey on students between the ages of 12 and 17 to find out the level of their nonmedical use or abuse of a variety of drugs, both legal and illegal.

Since our new regulations have been in place, we've seen a 50% or greater reduction in the proportion of students in high schools who are abusing these drugs. We think that's a massive and important contribution to stem the tide of drug abuse in the state.

Going beyond these points, we also looked at other data, for example, a Drug Abuse Warning Network showed that in New York State in the first year after the regulation was put in place there was a 48% reduction in drug overdoses. Also having looked at things like death certificates, we have seen a similar decline in the years following the regulations' implementation.

We also wanted to check physician's prescribing patterns to see if we'd restricted access to drugs such as benzodiazepines. We found that 90% of the physicians are still prescribing them, with no irregular prescribing patterns.

We also found that not all uses of benzos have gone down. For example, the use of diazepam (Valium), has actually more than doubled since it was placed on the triplicate system.

We also have responded to concern expressed by opponents of triplicate systems that the regulation might mean physicians would simply switch to drugs not on the triplicate system. That way, doctors could avoid the monitoring, but perhaps use older drugs which might suggest risk to patients.

But to the contrary, in 1992, three programs we monitored showed that the alternate drugs prescribed are back almost to the same level they were in 1989, a year before our regulation went into effect. In other terms, for every one hundred less benzodiazepine prescriptions we did not see more than a total of 20 new prescriptions for other drugs, and that was only in 1989. Simply put, physicians have chosen, as they have access to drugs with and without the triplicate system, to reduce significant overprescribing of benzodiazepines without having to resort to alternative medications.

What's even more telling is an indication of how triplicates do not interfere with legitimate prescribing for cancer pain. In fact, Morphine prescribing has gone up 1,500% since 1980. Clearly, physicians in the state feel free to prescribe these drugs when needed.

We've had criticism, too, about the triplicate system being archaic, producing mountains of paper. In terms of the triplicate itself, it is probably antiquated as a document. Today, electronic capture would be more efficient. But what's still good about our triplicate system is that we use a state-issued form with a serial number. Each document is a unique, traceable form. This fact alone has had tremendous value in stopping diversion.

For example, one of the common ways to obtain prescriptions illegally is for the abuser to copy or manufacture his own prescription pads and forge them. Our state-issued forms have serial numbers and special artwork in the background that makes it impossible to duplicate them. These are tamper-proof features. Since 1972, we've had only two attempts to copy the forms. Further, the dispensation of the state's forms is tightly controlled, available only to bonafide practitioners. In the end, we're led to conclude that we've had a very profound and long-lasting impact on a serious drug abuse problem in the state of New York.

■ ■ ■ ■ ■ ■

In contrast to the New York experience, in California where prescription fraud costs an estimated $1 billion annually, the triplicate prescription system does not receive high marks.

Dixon Arnett, Executive Director
Medical Board of California
Sacramento, California

When it comes to having a triplicate system, California needs to either "get on the ball" with it or get something that works. The triplicate system could work, but our system now is not effective. (California was the first state to implement a permanent triplicate system; it was adopted in 1939, as a result of the diversion of opiates.)

We have 103,000 physicians licensed by the state of California. That's nearly one-sixth of all physicians in the nation. About 77,000 are in active practice in the state. They issue a lot of prescriptions.

In Sacramento, the Hopkins Center houses two wings of the Department of Justice, wherein there is one of the most sophisticated, up-to-date, computerized criminal information systems in the world. But ironically, next door, is our triplicate system which has boxes and boxes and boxes of little slips of paper — prescription forms. The fact that this mountain of paper exists at all in today's age is bizarre. The system is a relic, a dinosaur.

Every day six employees take these prescription forms, one million a year, out of envelopes and stack them into piles and little, if anything, is ever done to them. The forms are supposed to be entered into a computer system, but the backlog is so great it takes forever to get the data entered into the computer.

We need to bring the system up to date. The good news is that the computer system which would handle this has existed for a long time. We could piggyback on the system. We could eventually even move into the use of "smart cards." This would be like having your entire medical history on a card like your driver's license. Doctors and pharmacists could read all your records immediately.

As far as the argument regarding loss of confidentiality with any monitoring system, I don't think it has merit. I think consumer protection outweighs concern about confidentiality.

■ ■ ■ ■ ■ ■

Meantime, California is actively considering the implementation of an electronic monitoring system, due in part, to the efforts of Sandra Bauer, a Sacramento business woman. Bauer's crusade against prescription drug abuse resulted from the death of her sister Jean, 35, a bank officer who died of an accidental overdose of Demerol in 1992. Bauer lobbied state legislators to convene the California Controlled Substances Prescription Advisory Council, which she then chaired during the council's one-year tenure.

"My sister was able to provide for her drug habit through the cooperation of licensed physicians and community pharmacies," Bauer says. "The prescriptions were written on the triplicate forms which are distributed to physicians in the state by the Attorney General's Office. And, private health insurance paid for all her medications," Bauer says.

An investigation into her sister's death came about only after she pushed for one. "Otherwise, she would have been buried and the case would have been closed." But following the investigation, the prescribing doctor, a 77-year-old heart specialist, was ordered to surrender his license to prescribe controlled substances and was put on five year's probation. The pharmacist was ordered to shut down his drug store for a month.

"Over time, my sister had received 10 times the normal number of prescriptions of the drug — a factor both the physician and pharmacist should have noted," Bauer insists. "If I hadn't complained to the medical board, the doctor who had prescribed numerous doses of Demerol and the druggist who filled the prescriptions would have gone untouched."

In the course of the advisory council's work, council members heard testimony on virtually all facets of prescription drug abuse and misuse in the state, including: chemical dependency, "accidental addicts," undermedication for pain, law enforcement issues, and triplicate and electronic monitoring systems. Topping the list of the council's recommendations: the implementation of an electronic monitoring system for all Schedule II-V drugs in the state.

If such a system had been in operation would it have saved the life of Bauer's sister? "Not necessarily, but my point is when a consumer gets a prescription filled, it appears that we have all kinds of tight controls. But in reality we don't; the clever con artists can get all the drugs they want. The current (triplicate) system simply doesn't work."

Pros and Cons of Triplicate Programs

The advantages and disadvantages of Multiple Copy Prescription Programs were recorded in a study, "A Review of Prescription Drug Diversion Control Methods," by the Bigel Institute for Health Policy, Brandeis University.

Advantages

- Targets diversion activities at patient, prescriber and dispenser level
- Includes all population groups in a state

■ Prevents or reduces prescription counterfeiting and alteration

Disadvantages

■ Somewhat burdensome to prescriber and dispenser
■ As currently implemented, does not include all prescribed controlled substances, and this is not comprehensive.
■ Data entry at state level is labor intensive

Electronic Monitoring

Electronic monitoring is often referred to as Electronic Data Transfer (EDT) or Electronic Point-of-Sale system (EPOS). To date, only a few states have adopted such a system to monitor dispensing of controlled substances.

Oklahoma became the first state to implement an electronic monitoring system. Considered the nation's best model, Oklahoma Schedule Two Abuse Reduction (OSTAR), went on line January 1990.

"I think it's working well. It's almost an invisible system," explains John Duncan, Chief, Diversion Division, Oklahoma Bureau of Narcotics and Dangerous Drugs. "That's why we haven't seen a change in the prescribing practices of most doctors. And really, we don't want to see that. We want to curb abuse, and not see legitimate patients go unmedicated."

Through OSTAR, pharmacists are required to enter Schedule II prescriptions — powerful drugs such as amphetamines, Dilaudid, Percodan and other narcotics — into the state's centralized, computerized data base. If such data is not submitted within 14 days of the point of purchase, civil penalties are imposed.

Information submitted electronically includes: Patient ID number (driver's license with photo ID); the National Drug Code, which tells the strength and form of the drug; date the prescription is filled; amount dispensed; pharmacy ID number and the physician's DEA number.

The mainframe data is analyzed by a private vendor, Argus Health Systems of Kansas City, Missouri; periodic summary reports show the state's prescription activity by categories including: geographic region; by physician, pharmacist or patient; and drug product. The reports also identify "outliers," in any of these categories showing questionable patterns.

A report is issued to the state Bureau of Narcotics. "If we have someone who goes to several different doctors and has several hundred tablets of Dilaudid, we can spot that immediately," according to Duncan. "It saves time and manpower. We make about 1,000 case inquiries annually. Without the computerized system, each case would take about eight hours of an agent's time. But now, with the stroke of a few computer keys, we can look at prescribing patterns and know if a problem really exists."

In the years since OSTAR's implementation, Oklahoma has seen a dramatic reduction in prescription fraud involving Schedule II drugs. The biggest reduction has come in the number of doctor shoppers and users of multiple pharmacies.

Though it's a model system, OSTAR is not without weaknesses. "The system is only as good as the information entered into it," Duncan says. "We've had a little trouble with pharmacies entering data, pharmacy codes and national drug codes."

Also, the system tracks only Schedule II drugs, and according to Duncan, that's created some new problems. "Now that the criminal element is aware that we're monitoring Schedule II drugs, they're moving into the Schedule III drugs, which include benzodiazepines, that are not monitored electronically at all; we have to search these manually. Unfortunately, the state does not have the legal authority or the dollar resources to begin tracking Schedule IIIs."

Another OSTAR limitation involves patient ID numbers. If the patient's driver's license number is used, the system can detect doctor-shopping or the acquisition of excessive amounts of controlled substances. However, if another ID number is used, for example, that of the individual picking up the prescription, the system's ability to detect diversion is lessened. Also, because ordinary paper prescription pads, not serialized or traceable, are used, OSTAR does not prevent forgeries.

The annual cost for operating OSTAR is under $200,000, considerably less than the projected $600,000 to run a state triplicate program.

In addition to Oklahoma, Hawaii and Massachusetts use EDT; other states are considering the implementation of electronic systems. Nine states are using partially automated monitoring systems.

Advantages and disadvantages of electronic monitoring, according to the Brandeis University study:

Advantages

- Targets diversion activities at patient, prescriber and dispenser level
- Not burdensome to prescriber
- Includes all population groups in a state
- Electronic entry speeds report generation

Disadvantages

- Somewhat burdensome to dispenser even for selected drugs
- Would be more burdensome to dispensers if all prescribed controlled substances were included
- Not all pharmacies are computerized

PART FOUR

Tools & Resources
for Recovery

14 Recovery...Taking the Journey Inward

While advanced technology, including electronic monitoring of prescription drugs, may curb illegal diversion of pharmaceuticals, personal recovery is far from being high-tech. Recovery is an affair of the heart and soul.

If you're starting recovery or are already underway, perhaps you've learned that the healing process requires a journey inward — coming to know, understand and love yourself in ways you never have before. Especially if this path is new to you, gaining some insights about the nature of dependency and your relationship with yourself and others can help you build a foundation for growth.

The following affirmations are offered with the hope that they may in some way enlighten you as you move along in your journey. These messages are not intended as a "cure-all," nor are they universal truths. Rather, they are the author's opinions, gleaned from his own life experience, his own journey. As they say in support groups, take what you like and leave the rest.

- **By understanding my past, I can better understand my needs today.**

  In childhood, we are totally dependent on our parents for physical and emotional nurturing. However, if abandoned either emotionally or physically by our parents, we can grow up with unmet dependency needs. Then, throughout life, we may experience feelings of emotional emptiness or "a hole in our hearts." Unmet dependency needs can be a catalyst for addiction or compulsive behavior. We sometimes turn to chemicals to fill the emptiness or to relieve painful feelings.

- **As I child, I did not choose to be hurt emotionally. Now, as an adult I can meet my own needs.**

  If you were abandoned in some way as a child, you were not responsible for it. Still, you may have blamed yourself for Mom's or Dad's actions. Children can't risk hating or rejecting their only caretakers, so they often turn the anger, even hate, inward toward themselves. But realize that a parent's choice was not your doing. Don't own it.

- **I am capable of leading a fulfilling life.**

  If we've experienced abandonment as children, later, as adults, we may find ourselves dealing with feelings of shame, depression, loneliness and low self-esteem. Many of us endure these feelings for decades, not realizing that healing and recovery is possible.

- **I can learn to experience a full range of human emotion.**

  Growing up, if we were faced with painful situations or feelings, we may have learned to numb feelings or pain as a way to protect ourselves. Unfortunately, we may still be numbing most of our feelings. Once we've numbed out, we're cut off from our inner feelings, our intuition.

- **I am learning to trust myself and others.**

  Trusting others does not come easily to those of us who have experienced abandonment or rejection from our primary caretakers.

■ **I am a valuable person.**

Growing up, if we were not affirmed, we did not feel valued. We came to believe that our feelings weren't important...that we were not important.

■ **I will build relationships with dependable people.**

Those of us who fear being abandoned often choose untrustworthy friends or mates who will eventually abandon us. If we recognize this pattern, we can stop it.

■ **I am learning what I need to do to take care of myself.**

We're never really "fixed," or totally cured from having unmet dependency needs. But if vigilant about taking care of ourselves, we can, indeed, be happy.

■ **I am developing healthy ways to cope with uncomfortable feelings.**

Compulsive behavior — that which we feel we cannot stop — is a mechanism for coping with anxiety. We might overeat, drink, do drugs, act out sexually, spend money or gamble...to ease the pain. However, we can never do enough of any of these behaviors to really fill the void we feel inside. And mostly, we end up feeling shame.

■ **I am rich with internal resources. I will use these resources to be less dependent on others.**

Have you ever felt addicted to a person, someone you can't live without, even if the relationship is not a "healthy" one? Usually, these people have struck in us some sort of primal chord, reminiscent of the love we felt for someone in our childhood. We may feel terrified of letting go.

■ **I realize that my feelings of powerlessness don't have to control me.**

Willpower is not the problem when it comes to stopping compulsive behaviors. We can demonstrate tremendous amounts of will in many areas of our lives and still feel powerless at times.

■ **I know the value of having balance in my life.**

Remember the acronym: H-A-L-T — hungry...angry...lonely...tired. Try not to let yourself experience these feelings to excess. They can trigger compulsive actions.

■ **I am willing to risk reaching out to others for my own well-being.**

Even though you may have been a loner, not likely to share your innermost self with others, find a support group or at least one other trusted person to whom you can eventually tell your life story, including all your secrets. Let the recovery begin.

■ **I realize that part of being independent is knowing when to ask for help.**

Support groups expedite recovery. They are an immense source of sharing, caring, understanding and comfort. Take yourself to several such meetings. Give the meetings a chance to work for you.

■ **Sometimes I must experience uncomfortable feelings in order to heal.**

Knowing intellectually about recovery doesn't accomplish enough. Recovery takes feeling the feelings and following up with actions.

■ **I am learning to respect myself.**

Recovery involves learning emotional boundaries, learning what's safe for me and what isn't it.

■ **I will demonstrate my love of self by doing nice things — big or small — for myself.**

It sounds trite, but a big part of recovery involves learning to love yourself. That doesn't mean being self-centered. It means learning to nurture yourself. Become a loving caretaker for yourself.

- **I do not need to be enmeshed in toxic relationships.**

As you recover from painful experiences and regain personal power, you may find yourself giving up certain friendships. As we become healthier, more balanced, we may find unhealthy relationships no longer fill a need for us.

- **I am unique, yet so much like everyone else.**

Once into emotional healing, you realize that you're like thousands of other people on the face of this earth, even though you may have thought no one else ever felt the way you did.

- **I understand the need for objective guidance in changing behaviors and attitudes. I am open to learning.**

People coming from abusive families don't know what normal is. Some think that pain and suffering is normal.

- **I will stop the buck here.**

Without intervention, education and effort to change, dysfunction in families is passed onto generation after generation.

- **I can recover...like many others have done.**

If you're discouraged about recovery, don't give up. Draw from the knowledge that millions have recovered from chemical dependency. They, too, felt hopeless at one time. Recovery is possible.

- **If I'm coping with the dependency of a friend or relative, I can love, yet detach from other persons enough to let them be responsible for their own behavior.**

If you're trying to rescue someone who's chemically dependent, you may be enabling him or her, inadvertently assisting him or her in continuing destructive behaviors. If you're always there to "clean up the mistakes," why should he or she change?

■ **I realize if my concerns over others' dependency are perceived by them as criticizing or "nagging," I'm not being supportive.**

It's very difficult to watch those you love do harm to themselves. If loved ones are refusing help or treatment, let them know you're there to help when they're ready. Unfortunately, you cannot do much for those who aren't interested in helping themselves.

■ **I can learn how I might be contributing to an unhealthy relationship.**

If you believe you're enabling, get help for yourself. Join a support group. Find out what you're deriving from being the rescuer.

■ **I deserve to live in a safe, nurturing environment.**

A loved one's chemical dependency takes a toll on the entire family. You are not responsible for the dependent one's actions. If your loved one won't make positive changes, perhaps you'll need to. Are you considering your own well-being, your own healing and recovery?

Resources

Center for Substance Abuse Prevention
Regional Alcohol and Drug Awareness Resources Network State Centers

Alabama

Division of Substance Abuse Services
Alabama Department of Mental Health/Retardation
200 Interstate Park Drive, P.O. Box 3710
Montgomery, AL 36193
(205) 270-4640

Alaska

Alaska Council on Prevention of Alcohol and Drug Abuse, Inc.
3333 Denali Street, Suite 210
Anchorage, AK 99503
(907) 258-6021; Fax: (907) 258-6052

American Samoa

Department of Human Resources, Social Service Division
Drugs and Alcohol Program
P.O. Box 5051
Government of American Somoa
Pago Pago, AS 96799
(684) 633-4485; Fax: (684) 633-1139

Arizona

Arizona Prevention Resources Center
Arizona State University
Box 871708 Arizona State University
Tempe, AZ 95287-1708
(602) 965-9666; Fax: (602) 965-8198

Arkansas

Bureau of Alcohol and Drug Abuse Prevention
Freeway Medical Center
5800 W. 10th Street, Suite 907
Little Rock, AR 72204
(501) 260-4506

California

State of California
Department of Alcohol and Drug Programs
1700 K Street, 1st Floor
Sacramento, CA 95841-4022
(916) 327-8447; (800) 323-0633; Fax: (916) 323-0633

Colorado
Colorado Alcohol and Drug Abuse Division
Resource Department
4300 Cherry Creek Drive, S.
Denver, CO 80220-1530
(303) 692-2930; (303) 692-2956; Fax: (303) 782-4883

Connecticut
Connecticut Clearinghouse
334 Farmington Avenue
Plainville, CT 06062
(203) 793-7971; Fax: (203) 793-9813

Delaware
Office of Prevention
Department of Services for Children and Youth
  and Their Families
1825 Faulkland Road
Wilmington, DE 19805
(302) 633-2682; Fax: (302) 995-8324

District of Columbia
D.C. Alcohol and Drug Abuse Services Administration
Office of Information, Prevention and Education
2146 24th Place N.E.
Washington, D.C. 20018
(202) 576-7315; Fax: (202) 576-7888

Florida
Florida Alcohol, and Drug Abuse Association Inc.
1030 E. Lafayette Street, Suite 100
Tallahassee, FL 32301-4559
(904) 878-2496; Fax: (904) 878-6584

Georgia
Georgia Prevention Resources Center
Substance Abuse Services
2 Peachtree Street, 4th Floor, Suite 320
Atlanta, GA 30303
(404) 657-2296; Fax: (404) 657-6424

Guam
Department of Mental Health and Substance Abuse
709 Governor Carlos G, Camacho Road
P.O. Box 9400
Tamuning, GU 96911
(671) 646-9260; Fax: (671) 649-6948

Hawaii
Coalition For A Drug Free Hawaii
Prevention Resource Center
1218 Waimanu Street
Honolulu, HI 96814
(808) 593-2221; Fax: (808) 593-2325

Idaho
Boise State University
Idaho RADAR Network Center
1910 University Drive
Boise, ID 83725
(208) 385-3471; Fax: (208) 385-3334

Illinois
Prevention Resource Center Library
822 S. College
Springfield, IL 62704
(217) 525-3456; Fax: (217) 789-4388

Indiana
Indiana University
Indiana Prevention Resource Center, Room 110
840 State Road, 46 Bypass
Bloomington, IN 47405
(812) 855-1237; Fax: (812) 855-4940

Iowa
Iowa Substance Abuse Information Center
Cedar Rapids Public Library
500 1st Street, S.E.
Cedar Rapids, IA 52401
(319) 398-5133; Fax: (319) 398-0408

Kansas
Kansas Alcohol and Drug Abuse Services
Department of Social and Rehabilitation Services
300 S.W. Oakley
Topeka, KS 66606
(913) 296-3925; Fax: (913) 296-0511

Kentucky
Drug Information Services for Kentucky
Division of Substance Abuse
275 E. Main Street
Frankfort, KY 40621
(502) 564-2880

Louisiana
Louisiana Office of Alcohol and Drug Abuse
P.O. Box 3868
Baton Rouge, LA 70821-3868
(504) 342-9352; Fax: (504) 342-3931

Maine
Office of Substance Abuse
Information Resource Center
State House Station #57, Stevens School Complex
Augusta, ME 04333
(207) 624-6528

NPNP Representative
Office of Substance Abuse
State House Station
Stevens School Complex
Augusta, ME (NOTE — ZIP?)
(207) 624-6500; Fax: (207) 287-4334

Maryland
Alcohol Drug Abuse Administration
Department of Health and Mental Hygiene
201 W. Preston Street, 4th Floor
Baltimore, MD 21201
(410) 225-6914; Fax: (410)333-7206

SALIS Representative
National Health Information Center
11426-28 Rockville Pike
Suite 310
Rockville, MD 20852
(301) 468-2600; Fax: (301) 468-6433

Massachusetts
Prevention Support Services
The Medical Foundation
95 Berkley Street
Boston, MA 02115
(617) 451-0409

Michigan
Michigan Substance Abuse and Traffic Safety Information Center
2409 E. Michigan
Lansing, MI 48912-4019
(517) 482-9902; Fax: (517) 482-8262

Minnesota
Minnesota Prevention Resource Center
417 University Avenue
St. Paul, MN 55103-1995
(612) 224-5121 or (800) 223-5833

Mississippi
Mississippi Department of Mental Health
Division of Alcoholism and Drug Abuse
1101 Robert E. Lee Building, 9th Floor
239 N. Lamar Street
Jackson, MS 39207
(601) 359-1288

Missouri
Missouri Division of Alcohol and Drug Abuse
1706 Elm Street
P.O. Box 687
Jefferson City, MO 65102
(314) 751-4942; Fax: (314) 751-7814

Montana
Department of Institutions
Chemical Dependency Bureau
1539 11th Avenue
Helena, MT 59620
(406) 444-2878

Nebraska
Division on Alcohol and Drug Abuse
P.O. Box 94728
Lincoln, NE 68508
(402) 474-0930; Fax: (402) 474-1992

Alcoholism and Drug Abuse Council of Nebraska
650 J Street, Suite 215
Lincoln, NE 68508
(402) 474-1992; Fax: (402) 474-0323

Nevada
Bureau of Alcohol and Drug Abuse
505 E. King Street
Suite 500
Carson City, NV 89710
(702) 687-4790; Fax: (702) 687-5980

New Hampshire
New Hampshire Office of Alcohol
    and Drug Abuse Prevention
State Office Park, South
105 Pleasant Street
Concord, NH 03301
(603) 271-6100; Fax: (603) 217-5051

New Jersey
New Jersey State Department of Health
Division of Alcoholism and Drug Abuse
129 E. Hanover Street, CN362
Trenton, NJ 08625-0362
(609) 984-6961; Fax: (609) 292-3816

New Mexico
Department of Health/BHSD-DSA
190 St. Francis Drive, Room N3200
Santa Fe, NM 87502-6110
(505) 827-2601; Fax: (505) 827-0097

New York
New York State Office of Alcoholism
    and Substance Abuse Services
450 Western Avenue
Albany, NY 12203-3526
(518) 474-3460; Fax: (518) 485-2062

North Carolina
North Carolina Alcohol and Drug Resource Center
5109 University Drive
Durham, NC 27707-3703
(919) 493-2881; Fax: (919) 493-9392

North Dakota
North Dakota Prevention Resource Center
North Dakota Division of Alcohol and Drug Abuse
1839 E. Capitol Avenue
Bismark, ND 58501-2152
(701) 224-3603; Fax: (701)224-3008

Ohio
Ohio Department of Alcohol
    and Drug Addiction Services
2 Nationwide Plaza
280 N. High Street, 12th Floor
Columbus OH 43216-2537
(614) 466-6379

Oklahoma
Oklahoma State Department of Mental Health
and Substance Abuse Services
1200 N.E. 13th Street, 2nd Floor
P.O. Box 53277
Oklahoma City, OK 73117
(405) 271-8755; Fax: (405) 271-7413

Oregon
Oregon Prevention Resource Center (OPRC)
Office of Alcohol and Drug Abuse Programs
Oregon Department of Human Services
500 Summer Street
Salem, OR 97310-1016
(503) 945-5763 or (800) 237-7808; Fax: (503) 378-8467

Pennsylvania
PENNSIAC
Columbus Square
652 W. 17th Street
Erie, PA 16502
(814) 459-0245; Fax: (814) 453-4714

Puerto Rico
Administracion de Servicios de Salud Mental Y
Contra la Addicion
P.O. Box 21414
San Juan, PR 00928-1414
(809) 767-5990; Fax: (809) 751-5231

Rhode Island
Rhode Island Department of Substance Abuse
P.O. Box 20363
Cranston, RI 09290
(401) 464-2380
(800) 974-1111; Fax: (401) 464-2089

South Carolina
South Carolina Commission on Alcohol and Drug Abuse
The Drug Store Information Clearinghouse
3700 Forest Drive, Suite 300
Columbia, SC 29204
(803) 734-9559

South Dakota
South Dakota Division and Substance Abuse
3800 E. Highway 34
C/O 500 E. Capitol
Pierre, SD 57501-5070
(605) 773-3123; Fax: (605) 773-5483

Tennessee
Tennessee Alcohol and Drug Association
Statewide Clearinghouse
545 Mainstream Drive, Suite 404
Nashville, TN 37228
(615) 244-7066; (800) 889-9789; Fax: (615) 255-3704

Texas
Texas Commission on Alcohol
  and Drug Abuse Resource Center
710 Brazos Street
Austin, Texas 78701
(512) 867-8821; Fax: (512) 480-0679

Utah
Utah State Division of Substance Abuse
120 N. 200 West, 4th Floor
Salt Lake City, UT 84145-0500
(801) 538-3939

Vermont
Office of Alcohol and Drug Abuse Programs
103 E. Main Street
Waterbury, VT 05671-1701
(802) 241-2178; Fax: (802) 244-8103

Virgin Islands
Marcia Jameson
Division of Mental Health
Prevention Unit
#6 & 7 Estate Diamond Ruby
Charles Harwood Hospital
Richmond St., Croix, VI 00820
(809) 774-7700; Fax: (809) 774-4701

Virginia
Virginia Department of Mental Health
Office of Prevention
P.O. Box 1797
Richmond, VA 23214
(804) 371-7564; Fax: (804) 371-6179

Washington
Washington State Substance Abuse Coalition
(WSSAC)
12729 N.E. 20th, Suite 18
Bellevue, WA 98005-1906
(206) 637-7011; Fax: (206) 637-7012

West Virginia
West Virginia Library Commission
RADAR Network Clearinghouse
Cultural Center
Charleston, WV 25315-0620
(304) 558-2044; (800) 642-9021; Fax: (304) 348-2044

Wisconsin
Wisconsin Clearinghouse
University Health Services
1552 University Avenue
Madison, WI 53705
(608) 263-2797; Fax: (608) 262-6346

Wyoming
Wyoming Care Center
University of Wyoming
McWhinnie Hall, Room 115
P.O. Box 3374
Laramie, WY 82071-3374
(307) 766-1119

Resource & Information Agencies

Narcotics Anonymous (NA)
World Service Office, Inc.
P.O. Box 9999
Van Nuys, CA 91409
Ph. (818) 780-3951
FAX (818) 785-0923
Internet zoom@cerf.net
CompuServe 70700,2647

Mission
NA is a nonprofit, international community-based organization for recovering addicts. NA members learn from one another how to live drug-free and recover from the effects of addiction in their lives. The focus is on addiction rather than specific drugs. Founded in 1953 in Southern California by several drug addicts who wanted to stop using drugs, NA now has 22,000 groups in the United States, Canada and 53 other countries.

Services
NA Meetings
Referrals to local meetings (Call (212) 870-3400)
Complimentary group starts kits
Literature in several languages

Publications
Narcotics Anonymous, a basic text
The *NA Way Magazine*, monthly subscription
Newsline, general information from the NA Office
Meeting by Mail, newsletter for addicts isolated by
   location or circumstance
NA Update — A newsletter for professionals
Various other pamphlets

Alcoholics Anonymous (AA)

General Service Office of Alcoholics Anonymous
P.O. Box 459
Grand Central Station
New York, NY 10163
(212) 870-3400; (212) 647-1680 — Meeting Referral Line,
   for information about AA meetings worldwide.

Mission

Alcoholics Anonymous is a fellowship of men and women to share their experience, strength and hope with each other that they may solve their common problem and help others recover from alcoholism.

AA is an informal society of more than 2,000,000 recovered alcoholics in the United States, Canada, and 134 other countries. These men and women meet in local groups, which range in size from a handful in some localities to many hundreds in larger communities.

Services

AA meetings
Twelve step recovery program
Local and national referral services to local groups.

Publications

Alcoholics Anonymous widely known as the "Big Book," *The Twelve Steps* and *Twelve Traditions* also known as the "12 and 12." Various other books, pamphlets, and audio-visual materials.

American Pharmaceutical Association
2215 Constitution Avenue NW.
Washington, DC 20037-2985
(202) 628-4410
FAX (202) 783-2351

Mission

The American Pharmaceutical Association (APhA) is a professional organization of pharmacists and specialists who know the chemical make-up and correct use of medicines. Pharmacists dispense drugs according to formal instructions given by doctors, dentists, or podiatrists and can answer questions about non-prescription products sold in pharmacies.

Services

The Association offers continuing education programs for pharmacists.

The Long-Term Care Section focuses on the needs of pharmacists who work in nursing homes, home care agencies, and hospices.

The APhA Foundation distributes health information to the general public.

Publications

APhA Pharmacy Today is distributed to approximately 100,000 pharmacists. *The Journal of Pharmaceutical Sciences* and *American Pharmacy* are published monthly. Materials for the public include the National Medical Awareness Test and the Self-Medication Awareness Test. A list of publications is available on request.

American Psychiatric Association

1400 K Street NW
Washington, DC 20005
(202) 682-6239

Mission

The American Psychiatric Association is a professional society of psychiatrists, medical doctors who specialize in treating individuals with mental or emotional disorders.

Services

The Association supports research to improve the diagnosis, treatment and rehabilitation of individuals with mental or emotional illness, sets standards for facilities that provide psychiatric care, and offers continuing education programs for psychiatrists.

The APA's Council on Aging evaluates care for older patients and offers training programs in geriatric psychiatry. Issues of particular concern include the use of medicines by older people, nursing home care, and treatment of patients with Alzheimer's disease and other dementias.

Individuals can contact the Association to locate a psychiatrist for consultation.

Publications

The American Journal of Psychiatry and the *Journal of Hospital and Community Psychiatry* are published monthly. *Psychiatry News* is distributed twice a month to members.

The American Psychological Association
1200 17th Street NW
Washington, DC 20036
(202) 955-7600

Mission

The American Psychological Association (APA) is a professional society of psychologists, health professionals who counsel people with mental, emotional, or behavioral problems.

Services

The Association offers continuing education programs for psychologists, establishes professional qualifications, and supports mental health research.

The Division of Adult Development and Aging conducts research on the psychosocial aspects of aging.

PsychAbstracts, a computerized database, provides references to journals, books, technical reports, and other publications dealing with psychology.

State chapters help individuals locate a psychologist for consultation and investigate complaints about individual counselors .

Publications

Psychology and Aging is published quarterly. *Psychology Today* and *APA Monitor* are distributed monthly. A number of brochures about mental health are available to the public.

American Society of Addiction Medicine

4601 North Park Avenue, Suite 101
Chevy Chase, Maryland 20815
Ph. (301) 656-3920

Mission

The American Society of Addiction Medicine is an international association of 3,000 physicians dedicated to improving the treatment of alcoholism and other addictions; ASAM endeavors to educate physicians and medical students, promote research and prevention and enlighten and inform the medical community and the public about these issues.

Services

The Annual Medical-Scientific Conference
The Ruth Fox (Founder) Course
The Medical Conference on Adolescent Addictions
The Medical Review Officer (MRO) Training Course
The Conference on Nicotine Dependence
Review Course
The State of the Art Course

Publications

Journal of Addictive Diseases
Principles of Addiction Medicine (1994)
ASAM Patient Placement Criteria (1991)
Review Course Syllabus (1990)
AIDS Guidelines for Facilities
ASAM News
ASAM Health Care Alert
Addiction Medicine
Fellowships Guidelines (1992)
Ruth Fox Course Syllabus (1993 & 1994)

Benzodiazepine Anonymous (B.A.)

6333 Wilshire Blvd., Suite 506
Los Angeles, CA 90048
(310) 652-4100

Mission

B.A. helps individuals withdraw from and live free of the use of benzodiazepine drugs. B.A. offers help in the form of associations with persons who have had similar dependency experiences. Members listen, ask, and share. B.A. has groups in the Los Angeles area.

Services

Regular support group meetings.

A twelve step program of recovery.

Publications

Benzodiazepine Anonymous Twelve Steps and an information sheet "Benzodiazepine Anonymous: Why We Are Here?"

Center for Substance Abuse Prevention (CSAP)

5600 Fishers Lane
Rockville, MD 20857
(301) 443-9936
FAX (301) 443-5592

Mission

The Center for Substance Abuse Prevention (CSAP) provides national leadership in the federal effort to prevent alcohol, tobacco, and other drug problems which have been linked to other serious national problems: crime and violence, rising health care costs, school failure, HIV/AIDS, teen pregnancy, and low work productivity.

Services

CSAP funds demonstration grants, operates a national prevention training system, produces a wide array of information and educational tools, manages a national clearinghouse, and operates resource centers and telephone helplines.

Resource Centers

The National Clearinghouse for Alcohol and Drug Information is the nation's central clearinghouse for materials on all aspects of substance abuse. Call 1-800-729-6686.

The National Resource Center for the Prevention and Treatment of Alcohol, Tobacco and Other Drug Abuse and Mental Illness in Women (the Women's Center). Call 1-800-354-8824.

The National Volunteer Training Center for Substance Abuse Prevention. Call (703) 931-4144.

The National Center for the Advancement of Prevention. Call (301) 443-7942.

Publications

Prevention Pipeline, a bi-monthly periodical and 150 other resource publications.

Food and Drug Administration

5600 Fishers Lane
Rockville, MD 20857
(301) 443-3170

Mission

The Food and Drug Administration (FDA) establishes Federal Government regulations concerning the safety and effectiveness of food products and additives, human and veterinary drugs, cosmetics, products that emit radiation, and medical devices.

Services

The Office of Consumer Affairs answers questions about the side effects, safe use, and effectiveness of vitamins, drugs, cosmetics, medical devices, and products that produce radiation (x-rays, microwaves, lasers, sound waves, ultraviolet radiation, and infrared radiation).

The FDA approves drugs used in the United States and supports research on the health effects of radiation exposure.

The FDA enforces the Food, Drug, and Cosmetic Act and related laws to protect consumers from unsafe and impure foods, drugs, and cosmetics.

Publications

Free publications include *Tuning in on Hearing Aids, Are Routine Chest X-rays Really Necessary?, Get the Picture on Dental X-rays, The Big Quack Attack, Medical Devices*; as well as material on nutrition and drug labeling. *FDA Consumer* is published monthly.

National Committee on the Treatment of Intractable Pain

P.O. Box 9553
Friendship Station
Washington, DC 20016
(202) 965-6717

Mission

The National Committee on the Treatment of Intractable Pain is a nonprofit organization that promotes education and research on the prevention and treatment of pain. The Committee relies on the expertise of professional advisors in medical, legal, bioethical, psychological, and religious fields.

Services

The Committee collects information about effective methods of pain control and pain research and makes this information available to health professionals and the general public.

Publications

A newsletter is published quarterly. The Committee also distributes a number of articles on pain research. A list of materials is available on request.

National Council on Alcoholism
7th Floor
12 West 21st Street
New York, NY 10010
(212) 206-6770

Mission
The National Council on Alcoholism, a private, nonprofit organization, works to educate the public about the disease of alcoholism.

Services
The Council distributes information about alcoholism to the general public and health professionals.

Local chapters around the country offer community service programs to educate the public about alcoholism and to help alcoholics and their families.

Technical assistance is provided to community organizations seeking to identify groups of people at risk of becoming alcoholics and to develop programs to meet the needs of these individuals.

The Council also maintains a comprehensive library of materials on alcoholism.

Publications
The Council offers print and audio-visual materials. Pamphlets especially for older people include *Older People and Alcoholism, Substance Abuse Among the Elderly,* and *The Unseen Alcoholics—The Elderly.* A list of materials is available on request.

National Council on Patient Information and Education

Suite 810
666 11th Street NW
Washington, DC 20001
(202) 347-6711

Mission

The National Council on Patient Information and Education, a nonprofit consortium of business, consumer, government, and professional groups, works to educate the public about prescription medications.

Services

Members are encouraged to develop public education programs.

The Council serves as a clearinghouse of information about existing national, state, and local medication information programs sponsored by member organizations.

A multimedia campaign is being developed to improve the use of prescription medicines by older Americans. This campaign will urge older consumers to talk with their doctor, nurse, or pharmacist about the uses and possible side effects of prescription drugs.

Publications

The Council distributes dozens of booklets, posters, pamphlets, media kits and a monthly newletter, *Talk About Prescriptions*. Other publications include the *Directory of Prescription Medicine Information and Education Products, Programs and Services* and *Approaches for Improving Prescription Medicine Use by Older Americans*.

National Institute on Alcohol Abuse and Alcoholism

5600 Fishers Lane
Rockville, MD 20857
(301) 443-1677

NATIONAL CLEARINGHOUSE FOR ALCOHOL AND DRUG ABUSE INFORMATION
1-800-729-6686

Mission

The National Institute on Alcohol Abuse and Alcoholism, part of the Public Health Service, is the Federal Government's principal agency for developing effective strategies to deal with problems and issues associated with alcohol abuse and alcoholism.

Services

The Institute conducts and supports studies of alcohol-related disorders and sponsors community surveys to assess the risks of alcohol abuse among various population groups.

Researchers funded by the Institute work to identify new ways to prevent alcohol abuse.

The National Clearinghouse for Alcohol and Drug Abuse Information provides information to health professionals and the public about the risks and consequences of alcohol and drug abuse.

Publications

Alcohol Health and Research World is published quarterly. The Institute also distributes pamphlets, books, and posters on alcohol abuse and alcoholism. A list of publications is available on request.

National Institute of Mental Health

Public Inquiries Office
Room 15C-05
5600 Fishers Lane
Rockville, MD 20857
(301) 443-4513

Mission

The National Institute of Mental Health (NIMH), part of the Federal Government's Alcohol Drug Abuse, and Mental Health Administration conducts and supports research to learn more about the causes, prevention, and treatment of mental and emotional illnesses.

Services

NIMH-supported researchers in hospitals, universities, and mental health centers around the country are studying biological, genetic, psychological, social, and environmental factors related to mental health and mental illnesses.

The Mental Disorders of the Aging Program specializes in research to learn how the aging process affects mental health and mental illness.

The Institute collects and distributes scientific and technical information related to mental illness, as well as educational materials for the general public.

Publications

Free publications include *Depression in the Elderly, Senile Dementia, Useful Information About Alzheimer's Disease, Plain Talk About Aging, Plain Talk About Handling Stress,* and *Care of the Mentally Ill in Nursing Homes.* A list of materials is available on request.

National Library of Medicine

8600 Rockville Pike
Bethesda, MD 20894
(301) 496-5501

MEDLARS SERVICE DESK
1-800-638-8480 (outside Maryland)
(301) 496-6193 (for residents of Maryland)

Mission

The National Library of Medicine (NLM), part of the National Institutes of Health, is the world's largest medical research library containing more than 3.5 million journals, technical reports, books, photographs, and audio-visual materials covering more than 40 biomedical and related subjects.

Services

Materials may be consulted at NLM or borrowed through interlibrary loan.

References to the most current indexed journal articles by subject area can be retrieved quickly through the MEDLARS databases. These databases include biomedical journals, audio-visual materials, hospital and health care literature, toxicology information, medical ethics information, cancer literature, history of medicine literature, and publications on reproductive biology.

Seven Regional Medical Libraries coordinate regional activities handling requests for health literature not available locally to the NLM.

Information specialists at the MEDLARS Service Desk answer questions about searching the MEDLARS databases.

Publications

Publications include *MEDLARS: The World of Medicine at Your Fingertips*, fact sheets about the programs and services of the library, and a list of Regional Medical Libraries.

U.S. Pharmacopeial Convention

12601 Twinbrook Parkway
Rockville, MD 20852
(301) 881-0666

PUBLICATIONS ORDERING SERVICE
1-800-227-8772 (toll-free)

Mission

The U.S. Pharmacopeial Convention (USPC) is a nonprofit corporation that sets standards of strength, purity, packaging, and labeling for medical products used in the U.S.

Services

The USPC provides information to health professionals and the general public about almost all drugs available in the United States including a description of the medicine and information about its proper use and possible side effects.

Health professionals may call the USPC to report improper drug labeling, defective components, performance failures poor packaging, and incomplete or confusing instructions.

Publications

Public education materials include *About Your Blood Pressure Medicines* and *About Your Medicines*. The USPC also publishes *USP Dispensing Information* (USPDI); Volume I contains drug use information in technical language for health care providers and Volume II is written especially for patients.

Bibliography

Chappel, John, N. "Educational Approaches to Prescribing Practices and Substance Abuse." *Journal of Psychoactive Drugs* 23 (October 1991): 359-362.

Colorado Prescription Drug Abuse Task Force. "Drug Diversion Scenarios, Scams," Denver, Colorado, 1992.

Controlled Substances Advisory Council, *Proceedings of September 23, 1993.* Sacramento, California.

Cooper, James, R.; Dorynne J. Czechowicz; Robert C. Petersen; Stephen P. Molinari. "Prescription Drug Diversion Control and Medical Practice." *Journal of the American Medical Association* 268 (September 1992): 1306-1310.

DuPont, Robert L. "Benzodiazepines, Addiction and Public Policy." *New Jersey Medicine* 90 (November 1993): 823-826.

DuPont, Robert L. "Choosing the Right Treatment for the Patient with Anxiety." 60 *Modern Medicine* (April 1992): 64-76.

DuPont, Robert L. "Medicines and Drug Testing in the Workplace." *Journal of Psychoactive Drugs* 22 (October 1990): 451-459.

"Final Report of the Controlled Substances Prescription Advisory Council to the Legislature and the Attorney General," by Robert Presley. Sacramento, California, 1993.

"Final Report to the National Institute on Drug Abuse, a Review of Prescription Drug Diversion Control Methods," by Constance Horgan; Jeffrey Prottas; Christopher Tompkins; Linda Wastila; Melissa Bowden. Brandeis University, 1991.

Goldman, Brian; Craig Sinkinson; William P. Egherman; Greg Wokersien. "Unmasking the Illicit Drug Seeker, a Guide for Pharmacists." CME-TV, Hagerman, Idaho, 1993.

Hughes, Patrick H.; DeWitt C. Baldwin; David V. Sheehan; Scott Conard; Carla L. Storr. "Resident Physician Substance, by Specialty." *American Journal of Psychiatry* 149 (October 1992): 1348-1354.

Hughes, Patrick H.; Nancy Brandenburg; DeWitt C. Baldwin, Jr.; Carla L. Storr; Kristine M. Williams; James C. Anthony; David V. Sheehan. "Prevalence of Substance Use Among US Physicians." *Journal of the American Medical Association* 267 (May 1992) 2333-2339.

Joranson, David E.; Charles S. Cleeland; David E. Weissman; Aaron M.Gilson. "Opioids for Chronic Cancer and Non-Cancer Pain: A Survey of State Medical Board Members." *Federal Bulletin: The Journal of Medical Licensure and Discipline.* (June 1992): 15.

Joranson, David E.; Aaron M. Gilson. "Policy Issues and Imperatives in the Use of Opioids to Treat Pain in Substance Abusers." *The Journal of Law, Medicine & Ethics* 22 (Fall 1994): 215-223.

Lurie, Peter; Philip R. Lee. "Fifteen Solutions to the Problems of Prescription Drug Abuse." *Journal of Psychoactive Drugs* 23 (October 1991): 349-356.

Marcantonio, Edward R.; Gergory Juarez; Lee Goldman; Carol M. Mangione; Lynne E. Ludwig; Leonard Lind; Nathaniel Katz; E. Francis Cook; John Orav; Thomas H. Lee. "The Relationship of Postoperative Delirium With Psychoactive Medications." *Journal of the American Medical Association* 272 (November 1994): 1518-1522.

Pelton, Chet; Richard M. Ikeda. "The California Physicians Diversion Program's Experience with Recovering Anesthesiologists." *Journal of Psychoactive Drugs* 23 (October 1991): 427-430.

Prescribing Controlled Drugs. American Medical Association Informal Steering Committee on Prescription Drug Abuse. Joseph H. Skom, Chairman. Chicago, 1986.

Ray, W.A.; M.R. Griffin; W. Schaffner; D.K. Baugh; L.J. Melton. "Psychotropic Drug Use and the Risk of Hip Fracture." *New England Journal of Medicine* 316 (1987): 363-369.

Schwartz, Harold I., ed. *Psychiatric Practice Under Fire.* American Psychiatric Press, Inc. Washington, D.C. (1994).

Smith, David E., and Wesson, Donald, R. "Benzodiazepines and Other Sedative Hypnotics." *Textbook of Substance Abuse Treatment.* American Psychiatric Press, Inc. Washington, D.C. (1994): 179-190.

Troy, Mike. "Dealing with Diversion." *Drug Store News* 16 (September 1994): 1-6.

U.S. Department of Health and Human Services. Agency for Health Care Policy and Research. *Management of Cancer Pain: Adults,* by A. Jacox; D.B. Carr R. Payne., et al. Number 9. Washington, D.C.: Government Printing Office, 1994.

U.S. Department of Health and Human Services. Agency for Health Care Policy and Research. *Acute Pain Management in Adults: Operative Procedures,* by Daniel B. Carr et al. Number 92-0020. Washington, D.C.: Government Printing Office, 1993.

U.S. Department of Health and Human Services. Substance Abuse and Mental Health Services Administration. *Preliminary Estimates fromthe 1993 National Household Survey on Drug Abuse.* Advance Report Number 7, 1994.

U.S. General Accounting Office. *Report to Congressional Requesters on Medicaid Drug Fraud, Federal Leadership Needed to Reduce Program Vulnerabilities,* 1993.

Weintraub, Michael; Satesh Singh; Louise Byrne; Kumar Maharaj; Laurence Guttmacher. "Consequences of the 1989 New York State Triplicate Benzodiazepine Prescription Regulations." *Journal of the American Medical Association* 226 (November 1991): 2392-2397

Wesson, Donald, R.; David E. Smith. "Prescription Drug Abuse, Patient, Physician, and Cultural Responsibilities." *The Western Journal of Medicine* 152 (May 1990): 613-616.

Wilford, Bonnie, B.; Joseph H. Deatsch. "Prescribing Controlled Drugs: Helping Your Patients, Protecting Your Practice." Medical Education Course, University of South Florida, Tampa (1993).

Wilford, Bonnie, B. "Prescription Drug Abuse: Some Considerations in Evaluating Policy Responses." *Journal of Psychoactive Drugs* 23 (October 1991): 343-347.

Wilcox, Sharon, M.; David U. Himmelstein; Steffie Woolhandler. "Inappropriate Drug Prescribing for the Community-Dwelling Elderly." *Journal of the American Medical Association* 272 (July 1994): 292-296.

Zweben, Joan Ellen; David E. Smith; Pablo Stewart. "Psychotic Conditions and Substances Use: Prescribing Guidlelines and Other Treatment Issues." *Journal of Psychoactive Drugs* 23 (October 1991): 387-394.

Newspapers

"Abuse of Painkillers, Diet Pills Can be Prescription for Addiction." *Hartford Courant.* 7 January 1990.

"Addiction's at Home in Affluent Suburbs." *Memphis Commercial Appeal.* 11 April 1990.

"America's Legal Drug Traffic Kills as Quickly." *Corning* (California) *Observer.* 11 May 1992.

"Death Spurred Quest for Truth." *The Sacramento Bee.* 9 June 1993.

"Dentists Get Wise to Addicts' Drug Scam Attempts." *Boston Herald.* 4 August 1991.

"Do We OD on What the Doctor Ordered?" *Bridgeport* (Connecticut) *Post.* 9 January 1994.

"Druggist Suspended After Narcotics Overdose Death." *Palm Springs Press-Enterprise.* 8 August 1992.

"Law Proposed to Curb Abuse of Prescriptions." *Austin American-Statesman.* 20 August 1990.

"License Hearing for Physician Delayed Again." *Palm Springs Press-Enterprise.* 19 March 1992.

"Many Abusers Finagle Prescription Drugs." *Norfolk* (Virginia) *Pilot.* 21 February 1990.

"Medicaid Report Shows Pattern of Drug Abuse." *Lexington* (Kentucky) *Herald-Leader.* 14 September 1993.

"Newest Narcotic Darling is Life-Numbing Opiate." *Orange County Register.* 8 August 1993.

"State Seeks to Shut Down Pharmacy Over Narcotics." *Palm Springs Press-Enterprise.* 14 February 1992.

"Prescription Drug Abuse Up Sharply." *Richmond* (Virginia) *News Leader.* 3 December 1991.

"Prescription Drug Abuse Worse Here." (Nashville) *Tennessean.* 6 August 1990.

"Prescription for Death: White-Collar Drugs." *The Sacramento Bee.* 5 February 1992.

"Regulators Draw Consumers' Ire." *San Francisco Examiner.* 9 March 1992.

"State Health Officials Say Abuse of Prescription Drugs Climbing." *Greenville* (South Carolina) *News.* 25 February 1990.

"State Cracks Down on Prescription Drug Addiction." *Reno Gazette-Journal.* 25 November 1990.

"Study Critcizes Elderly's Prescriptions." *Los Angeles Times.* 26 July 1994.

"'Tailgate' Medicine Sales Rampant in Ethnic Areas." *Los Angeles Times.* 9 October 1993.

"Utah Still 'Speed' Trap, Drug Report Declares." *Salt Lake City Tribune.* 19 November 1991.

"Vicodin: Rx for Disaster?" *Santa Rosa Press Democrat.* 18 October 1993.

Index

About the Author

A uthor/journalist Rod Colvin is the author of numerous magazine articles and two nonfiction books — *First Heroes*, Irvington Publishers, 1987, and *Evil Harvest*, Bantam, 1992.

A former counselor, Colvin holds an M.S. degree in counseling psychology and a B.A. degree in sociology.

Please send:

Prescription Drug Abuse: The Hidden Epidemic

____ Copies at $14.95 each =   _____

Nebraska residents add $ .75 sales tax   _____

Shipping & handling: $3.00 for first book
$1.00 for each additional   _____

Total Enclosed   _____

Name _____

Address _____

City_____ State_____ Zip_____

Phone (   ) _____

- -

(Please clip or photocopy above section)

Send check or money order to:
Addicus Books
P.O. Box 37327
Omaha, NE 68137
Or, order toll free: 1-800-35-ABUSE
(1-800-352-2873)

Quantity Purchases

Organizations, associations, corporations, hospitals and other groups may qualify for special discounts when ordering more than 24 copies of *Prescription Drug Abuse: The Hidden Epidemic*. Please specify quantity desired. Write or call Special Sales Department, Addicus Books, P.O. Box 37327, Omaha, NE 68137.